To Jill
/with
Ali xx
you are one
special lady
x

WHAT
THE F✕CK
JUST
HAPPENED?

A SURVIVORS GUIDE
TO LIFE AFTER
BREAST CANCER

WHAT THE F✖CK JUST HAPPENED?

A SURVIVORS GUIDE TO LIFE AFTER BREAST CANCER

JEN ROZENBAUM

J. Fox Press
Columbia, SC

Copyright ©2020 Jen Rozenbaum

All rights reserved. No part of this book may be reproduced in any form without permission in writing from the author. Reviewers may quote brief passages in reviews.

No part of this publication may be reproduced or transmitted in any form or by any means, mechanical or electronic, including photocopying or recording, or by any information storage and retrieval system, or transmitted by email without permission in writing from the author.

Neither the author nor the publisher assumes any responsibility for errors, omissions, or contrary interpretations of the subject matter herein. Any perceived slight of any individual or organization is purely unintentional.

Brand and product names are trademarks or registered trademarks of their respective owners.

1st edition Published 2020
J. Fox Press
ISBN: 978-1-948604-15-4
Library of Congress Control Number: 2020909744

Prepared for Publication by Write | Publish | Sell
writepublishsell.com
Cover Design: Fresh Design

*This book is dedicated to all the beautiful women
who lost their battles with breast cancer…
You are warriors and will never be forgotten.*

Table of Contents

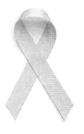

Chapter 1:
Reconstruction

re·con·struc·tion
rēkən'strəkSH(ə)n/

The action or process of reconstructing
or being reconstructed.
A thing that has been rebuilt
after being damaged or destroyed.

1

I FOUND MY CANCER IN A SELFIE. I sometimes wonder if I ever would have noticed it if I wasn't a photographer. In the image, I saw a shadow on my chest that I had never seen before, high above the nipple on the breastbone, just visible in my V-neck shirt. The mass was long, and it felt like a swollen muscle. I had always been taught to feel for a pea-sized lump, and this was not the size of a pea, nor was it a lump. I always had dense, cystic breasts. When I had my period, my breasts would swell, and I wouldn't feel the mass as much, so it would seemingly come and go, but it was still there, I later learned—just hiding.

"What do you think this is?" I asked my husband.

"It feels like a swollen muscle," he said.

"Yeah, it feels like that to me too." I had an appointment for a sonogram already scheduled in a few weeks, so I decided just to keep an eye on it and mention it at the appointment.

I live on Long Island, NY. The breast cancer rates are considerably higher here than in the rest of the United States, so because of where I live, combined with my dense and cystic breasts, I began getting mammograms and sonograms every six months once I turned forty. I had just been to the doctor a few months before to get a mammogram and sonogram, and the only thing they found were some small, seemingly harmless cysts. I wasn't worried. I take great care of myself, and there is no history of cancer in my family. Nothing would have made me think I would get breast cancer. Six weeks later, I was in my doctor's office for a sonogram to check the cysts that were previously found.

"Oh, hey, I almost forgot," I said to my doctor as we wrapped up my appointment. "Could you take a look at this?" I asked, pointing to what I thought was my swollen muscle.

The cysts were on the side of my breasts, but the lump was on my chest, outside the area the area they checked. The tech quickly spread ice-cold lubricant on the area in question. She started pressing my chest with the sonogram, and nothing came up on the screen—nothing. Then, she pushed *really* hard, and all of a sudden, I saw a football-shaped black hole on the screen, and I knew something was wrong.

The tech immediately ran to inform the doctor. My doctor came in to tell me that he was concerned, and he was not letting me leave without getting the mass biopsied. *What is happening? Do I call my husband? Should I be scared?* I thought. It was so far out of my mind that this scenario could happen. It was all a blur. After the doctor performed the biopsy and a subsequent mammogram, my doctor sat me down in his office.

"I want to warn you," he said. "I've been doing this for a lot of years, and I have seen a lot of things. I want you to be prepared for the worst."

My husband came right at the tail end of the conversation and asked, "If it's not cancer, what could it be?"

My doctor took a deep breath, looked at us solemnly, and replied, "There's nothing else it could be."

After my doctor's appointment, I spent two days not knowing for sure what was happening. I made a decision not to panic until it was time to panic. I stayed off Google. I figured that if it was cancer, life was going to change and quickly, so I just tried to keep myself busy and take care of as much as I could in those two days. I didn't cry. I didn't curl up on the couch. I just kept moving.

Two days later, I expected a call from my doctor with my test results. My husband took the day off work. The sitting home waiting was torture. Instead, we drove to a local town, walked around and did some shopping. We went to one of our favorite Mexican restaurants for lunch, and the second the food hit the table, my phone rang. I walked outside to talk to my doctor. I looked at my husband and shook my head – *yes* – and he went in to pay the bill and take our food to go. It was confirmed that I had invasive lobular carcinoma, a.k.a. breast cancer.

Cancer Is like a Tornado

In the weeks and months following, I had a double mastectomy and eight rounds of chemotherapy followed by breast reconstruction, twice. When I sat down to write this book, the word "reconstruction" kept coming to mind. It applies not only to my breasts but also to my post-cancer life. The first thing I did was look up the definition of reconstruction, and I couldn't help but chuckle to myself when I read, "A rebuilding of a thing that has been damaged or destroyed."

I liken cancer to a tornado; the similarities are many. A tornado touches down with little to no warning. It can level your home, your life, and your sense of security in the blink of an eye.

Certainly, you can hide from a tornado. You can go underground save yourself. In the same way of defense, you can treat cancer. You can have surgery, chemo, radiation, and whatever else the experts recommend. In both scenarios, you can take every action possible to secure your safety.

When the tornado passes, you emerge from the underground shelter and find your home in pieces. Some things are the same–you still have your friends and family. If you're lucky, you have a ton of support from those who care. However, when it comes down to it, all you want is to live in your house again. You want things to go back to normal, to sleep in your own bed, and to feel safe. You want your uncomplicated life back–but it's not there anymore. Everything has changed.

It's the same with cancer. When I was done with treatment, I saw familiar pieces of my previous life, but they didn't always make sense anymore. My safety, security, and normalcy were gone.

When I scheduled my mastectomy, I thought that was going to be the hardest part, but I made it through. When I began my first chemo treatment, I thought that would be the hardest part; again, I made it through. Don't get me wrong; they were both challenging and scary, but they didn't hold a candle to what was actually the hardest part of the process.

The Hardest Part of My Cancer Journey

The hardest part for me in this crazy journey has been reconstructing my life, my body, and my beliefs. After treatment ended, I was hit with the emotional shockwave of what my body had been through in the months prior.

I had panicked moments. The thought, *Holy shit, did I cut off my breasts?* would often hit my mind like a ton of bricks. Every now and again, someone would send me an article about how they are going to cure cancer, and it would make me mad. *Go figure*, I would think, *they are going to cure cancer after everything I just went through.* (Please note–I know this isn't a logical thought, and to be clear, I would be beyond exuberant for a cancer cure.)

When chemo was over, there were days when I felt moments of joy, followed by days where I shut my phone off and cried in bed for hours. It's hard for me to admit that, but it's also important for me to be honest about the process. Life after cancer is the hardest part; it's also the part that no one talks about–until now.

It's hard for me to admit the darkness, because as a survivor, so often I'm told, "You're a warrior–an inspiration; you are strong!" I *am* all of those things, but let's face it—I've been through hell, which sometimes makes doing and being those things more difficult than you can imagine.

The Difference Between Being Alive and Feeling Alive

When I finished cancer treatment, people asked me all the time how I was doing. I was struggling. I didn't want to lie and say I was great, but I also noticed that I was inadvertently shamed if I said I wasn't okay. I heard replies such as, "It could always be worse," or, "You should be grateful you are alive."

Those responses would always sting. They made me feel bad about myself. I *was* grateful to be alive, but cancer has taught me this invaluable lesson: there is a huge difference between *being* alive and *feeling* alive.

Saving your life is the goal of cancer treatment. I reached my goal, and I was incredibly grateful that I was alive. However, in doing so, I lost the feeling of being alive. Joy was often replaced with pain. Security was replaced with fear. I was living, but I was not alive.

You Are Stronger Than You Think

I remember heading into NYC one day for a follow-up appointment with my plastic surgeon. Sitting next to me in the waiting room was a woman who was about to see the doctor for the first time. She was newly diagnosed and was having a double mastectomy the following week. She and her partner sat patiently, working on a list of questions they needed to answer. I saw myself in her. Heck, I *was* her a short time ago.

We struck up a conversation, and I helped answer so many of her questions—questions that the doctor may know the textbook answer to but had no personal experience with. I gave her a list of what she would need to prepare; I explained the real timeline for recovery, and I was as honest as I could be.

She was scared and overwhelmed, just as I was when I was in her shoes. When the nurse called my name, I stood, put my hand on the woman's shoulder, and reassured her that she was going to be okay and that she could do it. It will be okay; she's stronger than she thinks.

I was sending that message to myself as much as I was sending it to her. Talking to her was a beautiful exchange of energy and reminded me how much I have been through and how far I have come. I am so grateful for that interaction. That beautiful woman unknowingly offered me some much-needed perspective.

Even though my physical self is now officially "reconstructed," I know there is more construction to be done, in the heart, the soul, and the mind. However, now, I can enjoy the process instead of dread it. Now, I focus on the rebuilding part instead of the damaged part. Rebuilding my life is a beautiful journey as I live beyond my fears, and the journey itself allows me to *feel* alive once again.

Let's face it, like it or not, cancer is now a part of our lives and thoughts every single day. I know you just want to go back to normal right now. I did too! Just as you were faced with choices about your cancer journey in the past, you are once again faced with a life-altering decision:

1. Stay where you are in your post-cancer, confused state, living a life that is consumed with stress, sadness, and anxiety, a lifestyle and mindset that is sure to decay your relationships, happiness, and worst of all, your health.

2. Or, take the steps you need to connect with yourself and reconstruct your mind, body, and soul. Doing this allows space for health, joy, and most importantly, normalcy in your life.

I know you want to feel normal again. I know because I have been in your shoes. I also know it's possible. I wrote this book to help you with the many layers of life after breast cancer, from the PTSD, to ridding yourself of toxins, to gaining back your femininity. I want you to know that you can put your life back together after a traumatizing life event. It's difficult, and it will change you, but your life can become better, brighter, and more beautiful through adversity. I can't tell you how excited I am that you picked up this book and that you are ready to go through this part of your journey. You have already taken the first step in the right direction.

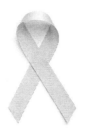

Chapter 2:
Embracing Struggle

*"The triumph can't be had
without the struggle."
— Wilma Rudolph*

2

BEING DIAGNOSED WITH BREAST CANCER in 2017 wasn't the first time I faced unexpected challenges in my life. In 2008, I was a stay-at-home mom to my beautiful daughter, Talia. My husband and I were in the process of trying to have another baby. I got pregnant pretty quickly once we started trying. At my twelve-week sonogram, we found out that the baby had no heartbeat and stopped growing around ten weeks. That led to a procedure and many following complications.

Once we were ready to try again, I once again got pregnant quickly, but at five-weeks pregnant, I suffered a life-threatening ectopic pregnancy and an emergency surgery. It was a time in which I found myself sad, frustrated, and alone. I was always the type to think positively and be optimistic, but I was struggling with my femininity and role as a mother. I felt I couldn't even protect my babies in my body. My thoughts were dark and overwhelming. I knew if I was going to survive that experience, I needed a distraction.

Photography as a Healing Tool

During that time, I first picked up a camera. I remember it clearly–it was a Nikon D80, and I had no idea what I was doing! I started by placing a glass on my coffee table and taking a photo. Then I moved a knob on the camera and took another photo. I did this for hours, moving knobs and taking pictures until I understood what the knobs did and how the camera worked.

Slowly but surely, I taught myself photography. In early 2009, I was invited by a photographer friend to assist her on a boudoir photoshoot. It was a chance for me to get out of the house and try something new, so I happily agreed. *What a life-changing day that was.* To this day, I am not sure I can explain why, but I knew in my bones that boudoir was my calling.

When I got home, I immediately started a boudoir photography business out of my house, and it took off like wildfire. *Spoiler alert: To my surprise, I also got pregnant with my second child just a short time later!*

Since 2009, I grew my business to include photography, teaching, public speaking, writing, and inspiring photographers and women throughout the world. I also used my skills and following to help heal others and myself through their breast cancer journeys through photography, videos, and now this book.

As I went through the journey of trying to have another baby, my spirit was shattered. My body and emotions took a beating. I cried often and hard. It was heartbreaking. I didn't understand it at the time.

However, hindsight is twenty-twenty. Looking back, it made complete sense. The timing wasn't right. I was put here for a reason, and if I had another baby when I wanted to and did not go through a life-changing struggle, I never would have discovered photography. If I never discovered photography, I wouldn't have a platform to reach women. If I didn't have that platform, I wouldn't have had the opportunity to spread awareness about breast cancer, and this book most certainly would not have existed.

This chain of events taught me multiple life lessons. As I mentioned before, I couldn't understand why I struggled with fertility, and I was equally confused, saddened, and shocked when I was diagnosed with breast cancer. I knew deep down that my struggle with fertility and the events that occurred after prepared me for my cancer journey. How? It proved to me that on the other side of struggle and pain are blessings and gifts. I learned that it's human to struggle. It's what you do with the struggle that counts.

From the minute I was diagnosed, I understood that having breast cancer was part of my purpose on earth. I knew that I had to go public and share the good, the bad, and the ugly. Without purpose, cancer was just an illness. With purpose, it was a platform for growth and change.

I want you to know that I write this book not from a place of superiority, but a place of solidarity. This chapter is meant to express to you how I solved the problem of not feeling normal after cancer, but here's the raw truth—I haven't completely figured it out.

You see, healing after a trauma like cancer takes time, and it's certainly not a linear process. Most days, I feel normal, even better than normal. I am killing it at life. I feel energetic, feminine, and healthy. There are still are days that exist in which I get sucked into the breast cancer black hole, and I find myself irritated, angry, and sad. Some days are filled with joy, and other days are filled with tears. The most important thing to know is that it is okay. Leaning into the emotions is part of the journey. Denying yourself of these emotions or fighting them only amplifies them. Trying to fight anxiety only makes you more anxious. Ignore your anger, and you will soon find yourself even angrier. Going through this process isn't about ridding yourself of all bad days. You will still experience bad days from time to time, but the more you lean into them, feel them, and then let them go, the more positive days you will have. This is what I found to be the key to getting your life back to normal—having more good days than bad and filling those good days with life, love, and hope.

I am almost three years out from being diagnosed with cancer. During those three years, I made videos and kept journals about my experience. This book is a compilation of those thoughts, my life experiences, tragedies, and triumphs that all led me to the process of reconstructing my life. Like my struggles with fertility, this struggle has also been a great gift I have been given, and I hope I can help you see it that way too.

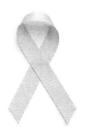

Chapter 3:
The Three Pillars of Wellness

*"Wellness encompasses a healthy body,
a sound mind and a tranquil spirit.
Enjoy the journey as you strive for wellness."*
— *Laurette Gagnon Beaulieu*

3

I HAVE MADE IT MY MISSION to cover as many topics as possible that are related to the ways life changes after breast cancer. First, I will guide you through defining and committing to a new normal. Then, I will share with you the actions I took to get me to my new normal, allowing me to live a more peaceful, joyous, and healthy life. These topics include areas within the three pillars of wellness: physical, emotional, and spiritual. Every topic I write about from self-care, training your brain and reconnecting with your femininity, etc. has physical, emotional, and spiritual components to them.

This book can be used in multiple ways. I recommend first reading the book cover to cover. Reading that way will allow you to understand the steps to this process from start to finish. You can follow the steps as you read them, or you can read the book without taking action, then go back, read chapter-by-chapter, and put the steps into action. I placed the chapters in the order that I recommend you do them. Often, one step is a prerequisite for the next one, but here's the beauty of this book: once you do all the steps, you are then able to go to any section you want at any time. Remember how I mentioned that this process isn't linear? This book is there as a reference any time you need it. There will be days you struggle to feel feminine for example; no problem, turn to Chapter 11 to refresh yourself on how you define femininity. If you struggle with negative thoughts, Chapter 9 will remind you how to flip the script in your brain.

This book is meant to help transform your post-cancer life in physical, emotional, and spiritual ways. A fulfilled, happy, healthy life of normalcy is easier to attain when three areas of life are in alignment with who you are.

Three Different Pillars of Wellness

Physical wellness is certainly high on our priority lists. Of course, physical wellness includes exercising getting enough sleep, and eating well. It also means making sure you are staying on top of doctor appointments, scans, treatments, etc. Developing healthy habits today helps build endurance and health to enjoy the life you are creating, as well as increasing your chances of a long life.

Emotional wellness includes being able to feel and express human emotions. The emotions include the full range, from negative to positive. It also includes having the ability to love and be loved and achieving a sense of fulfillment in life. Positive self-esteem, self-acceptance, and self-worth are also included in your emotional health.

Spiritual wellness involves your personal beliefs and values, which help give direction to one's life. Spiritual wellness encompasses a high level of faith, hope, and commitment to your individual beliefs, which in turn provide a sense of meaning and purpose. Being well spiritually means having the willingness to seek meaning and purpose in human existence, to question everything, and to appreciate the things, which cannot be readily explained or understood. Spiritually-well people seek harmony between what lies within as well as the forces outside themselves.

As you can see, these three pillars of wellness are key to reconstructing your life. When they are all in alignment, you will start feeling the normalcy you crave. When one, or more than one area, is out of alignment, that is when the bad days will sneak up on you.

Let me explain. Let's say that you physically feel great. You are working out and eating right. You have been doing spiritual work, meditating, and connecting to your breath. Things in the physical and spiritual areas of your life seem to be going smoothly. However, you experience nagging negative thoughts and fears you can't seem to control. That is an indication your emotional wellness is out of alignment, which is okay short term. However, if it carries on longer than that, it can bleed into your other areas of wellness. The negative thoughts could pop up during your meditations, making it difficult to focus. Sleeping at night is a challenge because the thoughts do not allow you to turn off your brain. This makes you tired and unable to work out the next day, and you find yourself grabbing comfort foods instead of your usual green smoothie.

It's not to say that our goal here is to achieve perfection every day; that's impossible. The key here is balance. Picture these three pillars as a three-legged stool. If one leg is a little off, it's okay; a wobbly stool can still support you. However, if a leg is broken, cracked, or unbalanced, you will fall on the floor.

As you go through the chapters of the book and apply what you learn to your life, always keep this trio of wellness in the back of your mind. In a moment you feel off-balance, all you need to do is identify which leg or legs are causing the problem. Some chapters are more heavily geared towards one pillar of wellness, and some incorporate all of them. Collectively, the chapters will help you heal all three areas and allow normalcy back in your life.

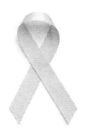

Chapter 4:
Re-Evaluate Your Life

"I'd rather regret the things I have done then the things I haven't done."
– Lucille Ball

4

Cancer is a horrible disease. Being diagnosed with cancer, no doubt, rocks your world. Because of that, you have the option of viewing it one of two ways:

1. Cancer ruined my life.
2. Cancer has given me a chance at a new life.

In a way, both perspectives are true, but the first statement comes from a negative point of view, and the second statement comes from a positive point of view. Since you picked up this book, and you are looking for guidance to rebuild your life, I can only imagine you have felt both ways. Cancer is evil, awful, and never welcomed in anyone's life. However, when we look at the aftermath of cancer from the second perspective, it becomes clear that cancer also brings gifts into your life, if you choose to find them.

Cancer both gifted me and changed my perspective of everything in my life. It changed me fundamentally, just as it changed how I view the world. Cancer made important things more important and unimportant things even less important. Because our perspective changes, so does how we view our lives. Therein lies the first step to this process: re-evaluating your life.

How to Re-Evaluate Your Life

The opportunity to re-evaluate your life is a huge gift wrapped in a big, red bow. Most people just live their lives day after day like Groundhog Day – going to work, taking care of kids, running errands, and paying bills. There's little joy or connection with oneself this way. Day after day goes by, and before you know it, life passed by, and you are left questioning what your legacy is.

Cancer woke me up to the fact that I don't want to live my life like that. Remember what I mentioned in Chapter 1? There is a significant difference between *being* alive and *feeling* alive, and I want to feel alive! I want to experience all life has to offer and leave a kick-ass legacy.

How do we live a life that we know will help us feel alive? Surely we still have to go to work, take care of the kids, run errands, and pay bills. How do we put our new perspective into place while still maintaining some normalcy?

The answer is simple. Before cancer, I lived my life forward, which is how most of us live. We are born, go through school, which prepares us to get a job, which prepares us to be adults and get married, and then we have children and raise those children to do the same. Next, we retire and hope to live long enough to run after our grandkids and do some traveling. Everything we do in life is to prepare for the next step.

There is validity to this way of living. Preparation and vision *are* important. I am not saying to disregard this way of life or thought process; it's important to be prepared. However, now I will tell you that I live my life backward first.

These days, I look at my life backward. I am not afraid of death; rather, I'm afraid of looking back on my life and feeling regret, so I continually ask myself, *what is it going to take to live the life I know I'm capable of living?* I live intentionally now, and I've embraced and enjoyed the process of putting my life back together the way I want it to be. Cancer is lonely and scary, but if we are fortunate, we also get a second chance at life. It's not enough to just be alive anymore; I want to live.

This second chance is a blessing and also frightening as hell. Finding balance is a struggle and one that the outside world may not understand. Ultimately, I believe that this second chance is a tremendous gift. We all have a limited amount of time on this earth. Let's live and reconstruct our lives in such a way that when we are at the end of our lives, we will look back knowing we were purposeful and gave it everything we had.

You may still be thinking, *backward?* Yes – *backward.* Another way to look at is by what I call the "deathbed principle." It's a morbid name, I know, but it's meant to shock you so that you won't forget it.

Let me explain. Take a moment, close your eyes and imagine yourself old and on your deathbed. You are surrounded by family and loved ones. You are all talking about reminiscing about life, laughing at memories, telling stories of events, and remembering the good and bad times. It's a beautiful time actually, surrounded by those whose lives you touched.

Then, one of them asks you, "Do you have any regrets in life?"

And there it is – the million-dollar question.

Do you have any regrets in life?

So, let me ask you right now, when you are on your deathbed, do you want to be riddled with regret or amazing memories, stories, and a legacy? I don't know about you, but I want to make decisions based on the deathbed principle and leave this earth with as little regret as possible. If you agree with me, just know you are in control of that narrative right in this moment. How exciting is that?

How to Live Life Backward

This is how I put the deathbed principle into place. When I find myself faced with making a decision about taking a risk or doing something out of my comfort zone, I ask myself a few questions, such as:

- Is this worth my time?

- How does this make me feel?

- Will this better me as a person?

- Is it worth the risk?

- Are my fears around this risk real?

- Will I regret it later if I say no?

Checking in with myself in that way assures that I find a balance between my average everyday life and a life that will be filled with memories and experiences. I have used this method to make seemingly small decisions and life-changing ones. This method came in handy when I decided to go on an amusement park ride with my kids that I would usually pass on (and loved it!). When I decided to train for a half marathon (even though I couldn't even run down the street without getting winded). It's also come in handy to make life-altering decisions such as starting a business, moving, or writing this book! These questions are a checkpoint to make sure I don't make rash decisions, but more importantly (and more commonly), they make sure fear doesn't get involved and hold me back from doing something amazing. My goal is to live in a balance between, you only live once (#YOLO) and being responsible. In other words, living a life balanced between looking forward and looking back.

If you are willing to see cancer as a gift, as I mentioned earlier in this chapter, honestly re-evaluating your life is the practice of opening that gift! Before you start journaling about what you think you want your life to look like, take a moment now and close your eyes. In front of you is a gift box. Get a clear picture in your mind what it looks like. Is it big or small? Is it beautifully wrapped? What color is the bow? Your precious new life is in that box, which means it deserves the most perfect wrapping possible. Now get curious, what's in the box? Picture yourself examining the gift. Pick it up. Is it heavy or light? Now give it a little shake. Do you hear anything? Ask yourself again, *what is in that box?* The only limit is your imagination. Now imagine yourself opening the gift and peeking inside. What do you see?

What you see is all the potential your life has to offer you. This is the perfect time to break out your journal and write down everything that is in the gift box. Just let the words and ideas flow. Don't limit yourself. Even if something seems far-fetched or unattainable, write it down. The more you can stretch your imagination, the bigger the gift. You have been through the trauma; now it is time to reap the benefits. That is the beauty of this second chance you have been offered.

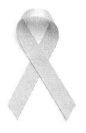

Chapter 5:
Commit to Yourself

"Unless commitment is made, there are only promises and hopes; but no plans."
– Peter F. Drucker

5

After I finished my cancer treatment, I started seeing a wonderful therapist. I went to her hoping to work through my feelings to heal post-cancer. She helped me in so many ways, and one of the pieces of advice she gave that I still refer back to often was, "Change comes only with great love or great pain." She was right! In fact, I will take it a step further and argue change can come from both great love *and* great pain existing in the same situation, at the same time.

You and I, we been through the great pain of cancer, and sometimes we still feel it. In this chapter, though, it's time to focus on some great love. Where will this love come from? It will come from you, of course. But love isn't enough to make your new life a reality. What needs to accompany your love is commitment.

Make a Commitment

Cancer can be a lonely and isolating disease. No matter how much support you have, how many loved ones come to chemo, or how many people cook you meals, it was you and you alone on that operating table. You, and you alone, were hooked up to the chemo. It doesn't mean that our loved ones don't experience their own journey and feelings; however, it does mean that we often find ourselves alone with our thoughts, fears, and challenges that no one else can understand. Because of this, you need to show up for yourself in a way you might not be used to in the following exercise. It might push you out of your comfort zone, and that's okay. I know for sure that you did hard things; you can do this too.

This is the part of the journey where you commit to yourself fully and truly. To reconstruct your life and feel normal again, it's vital that you take this step. This commitment means different things to different people, and this exercise is meant to guide you to find what it means to you.

In Chapter 1, I wrote about all the great things you can gain in your life by reading this book and putting it into action. Start by making a list of those things – all of them! I don't care if there are five things on the list or 5,000. In fact, I suggest not limiting yourself. Give yourself a period of time and just freely write. Ask yourself, *what do I have to gain if I commit to myself and reconstruct my life the way I would love for it to be?*

There are no right or wrong answers. You can go as deep or as shallow as you want to. This exercise is about you, your needs, and your own unique and beautiful post-cancer life.

Now that you have a list, it's time to sort the list into three categories: physical, emotional, and spiritual. As we discussed in Chapter 3, these are three pillars of your life, and they are the foundation of where reconstruction begins. I will show you an example from my list.

Things I have to gain by reconstructing my life:

Physical

I will have a healthier body.

I will have abundant energy and glow.

I will sleep more soundly.

Emotional

I will fear cancer less on a daily basis.

My PTSD will not get the best of me.

I will have closer relationships.

Spiritual

I will not stress over things I can't control in my life.

Meditation will make me calmer and more present.

I believe in something bigger than myself.

After you make your list, it's time to go back through your writing and assign the feelings that coincide with achieving that change. You may choose to do this for each item on your list or write down your feelings according to the category. Here are some examples:

Physical

I will have a healthier body – relief.

I will have abundant energy and glow – joy.

I will sleep more soundly – calm.

Emotional

I will fear cancer less on a daily basis – calm.

My PTSD will not get the best of me – in control.

I will have closer relationships – connected.

Spiritual

I will not stress over things I can't control
in my life – surrender.

Meditation will make me calmer and more
present – happy.

I believe in something bigger than myself – hope.

Now that you have a list of all the beautiful changes, life gains, and positive emotions that you see are available to you, it is time for you to write yourself a letter of commitment.

I love manifestation, and I use it quite a bit in my life. If you aren't familiar with manifestation and how to attract what you want in your life, here's a secret – you have already done it. That was exactly what the first part of this exercise was – manifestation!

Manifesting something in your life is as simple as knowing what you want and experiencing the beautiful feelings that come along with getting it. It may sound simple, and the truth is that it is. Where people usually fail in manifestation is that they forget to take action. Manifesting something in your life is not about sitting back, just hoping it shows up. Instead, manifestation is about knowing that you want something, believing you are deserving of the things that you want, truly feeling the feelings that come along with them, and taking action to make sure that what you want happens. This is why I often use the term "manifestaction;" manifestaction is a combination of manifestation and action.

That's where the letter to yourself comes in to play. This letter is your chance to get real with yourself. Nobody ever has to see this letter except for you, and that means you can let go of any worry that you will sound silly, be judged, seem egotistical or even batshit crazy.

What will you write in this letter? This letter is all about you committing to yourself. It's a chance for you to tell yourself that you believe in you. It's about reaffirming what you want in your new post-cancer life, the way you will feel in this life, and, most importantly, the actions you will take to get there.

Consider this letter a love letter to you, from you. Start with an abundance of compliments. I know this is hard for some people; if you are one of these people, take a moment to draw on the compliments other people have given you. Try to see yourself from an outsider's point of view. Remember that nobody sees this letter except yourself, so no compliment is too big or too small. You may feel drawn to include a list of all the difficult things that you've accomplished in your life, all of the victories in your life, and all the things you have to live for. In this letter, tell yourself that you are deserving of great love and a beautiful life. List all of the things that you are truly ready to commit to doing change your life. If you want to add more, add more. If you want to write less, write less. No matter how much or how little you write, I recommend your letter include these key points:

- Love and compliments from you, to you
- A reminder that you are deserving and capable of the life you desire
- A list of actions you are ready to commit to to make it happen
- All the ways your life will change (in all three pillars) after putting the list into action

Here are a few examples from my personal commitment letter:

Compliments: You are stronger than you know! You are a badass. You take tragedy and turn it into triumph. You love with all your heart. You are empathetic and care about others deeply.

Reminder: Jen, you are not only capable of creating the life you desire, but you are deserving of it. It's time to throw away your limiting beliefs. Believe in yourself so fiercely that no one can crush that belief with any words or actions. You are capable of things bigger than you can even imagine. Surround yourself with positivity and uplifting people and thoughts. Believe, believe, believe.

Actions: I will listen to my body and give it what it needs. I will push myself beyond the boundaries of what I think I am capable of. I will set healthy boundaries with people and events that I don't feel comfortable with and speak my mind when necessary. I will keep up with my doctor's appointments. I will continue to create content about breast cancer and be honest about my journey to help others who are walking in my shoes. I will be active five days a week. I will tackle any negative self-talk with words of affirmation.

How I will feel: Jen, when you keep this commitment to yourself, you will feel healthy emotionally, physically, and spiritually. When you are in alignment, you can accomplish so much. There was a peace you didn't have in your life before cancer. I commit to take these actions that will lead to peace, fulfillment, and joy.

This is only a small sample of the thoughts in my letter, but you get the idea. I chose to write it like an actual letter, but I also often incorporate bullet points for action items, compliments, and feelings. You can write a long letter or lists or keep them shorter. You know yourself best. Do you work better with having a long-term plan, or do you find that you work better by committing to one or two things at a time?

Personally, I work best by focusing on one thing, tackling that, and then moving onto the next. In my letter, I chose not to include more than a handful of actionable items at first. That's the beautiful thing about this letter; it's never done being written. It can always change, and as you grow, it should change. The most important thing is that at any given moment, you take action on the items you want to manifest in your life.

As Abraham Lincoln once said, "Commitment is what transforms a promise into a reality." This is not one of those low-level promises you are making yourself. I urge you to consider what you are promising yourself carefully, and I recommend you keep this letter handy. There are going to be a lot of times in life when your ego gets in the way of progress and, therefore, your new reality. When that happens, you will start hearing excuses rise to the surface. Your negative self-talk will be louder than usual. Your negotiation tactics with yourself will kick in. You may feel fear, doubt, and overwhelm. When you feel that way, it's a perfect time to pull out the letter, read it, and use it to remind yourself how awesome you are, how strong you are, and that you can do anything you put your mind to.

Let's be honest; you kicked cancer's ass. You can do this too.

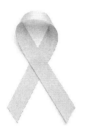

Chapter 6:
The New Normal

*"We are at our most powerful the moment
we no longer need to be powerful."*
— Eric Micha'el Leventhal

6

In the last two chapters, you spent time reevaluating your post-cancer life and making a commitment to yourself to take action on the changes you need to feel normal again. Now that the groundwork has been laid, it is the perfect time to address the word "normal" and working on accepting a "new normal."

You picked up this book because you wanted your life to go back to normal, meaning the way it was before cancer. I too wanted my life to go back to normal after cancer. I remember vividly telling my oncologist that no matter what happened, my treatment needed to finish by the end of December so that I could start the New Year off fresh. I recall telling myself over and over again that once treatment was over, I would go back to "normal."

After my last chemo session, I asked my husband to stop at Trader Joe's on the way home. I usually went straight home after chemo. This time I wanted to do something that I would do in my "normal" life, symbolic of the end of my treatment journey. As I walked into Trader Joe's, I remember thinking to myself that here I was, for the first time in a long time, just like everyone else. I was done with chemo, and I was normal again. As I went through the store, I was terrified of touching anything or anyone in fear of germs. I was tired, nauseous, and overwhelmed. I know logically, it was unrealistic for me to expect to walk out of chemo and into the grocery store and feel like myself. I was so unbelievably desperate to feel normal that I did it anyway. But it didn't feel normal, and I didn't feel anything close to normal. For a solid year, I spent every day waking up, praying, and hoping that was going to be the day that I felt like myself again.

Day after day, I was disappointed. Day after day, I felt like a stranger in my own life. I spent hours rummaging through old pictures of myself. I used to play this mind game where I would look at a photo and try to remember how old I was, comparing myself to the person back then. Was I fatter now, thinner now? Was my hair as full as it was back then? Did I have more wrinkles now? Did cancer age me before my time? Was I happy that day? Did I feel good? I used to think, *if I could just look like the Jen in those photos, I would feel like the Jen in those photos.* I obsessively looked at these old pictures, desperately wanting to go back to that woman.

I thought that by doing this, I could reconnect to myself. However, in actuality, all I was doing was causing myself pain. It wasn't until somebody said to me one day, "Jen, even if you didn't have cancer, you would never be that person again. We are all changing every day, and you are no exception to that rule. Embrace who you are today because tomorrow you will surely be different too."

I can't lie. Sometimes I still find myself looking back at old photos, longing for my pre-cancer days. The truth is, though, that when I do that now, I don't recognize the woman I see. It's almost as If I am looking at photos of a stranger. I am not that person anymore, and I never will be again. I remind myself every time I feel that pit in my stomach of wanting to be that girl that I am a stronger, wiser, more badass woman now, and who I am is the new normal. I am proud of who I am now. Even though, in my mind, I created the story that I was happier before cancer, it's not true. Pre-cancer life came with its own set of challenges. I just convinced myself that life before cancer was great, and life after would never be the same. I knew that had to change.

The Art of Surrendering

How did I change my old thinking habits and get comfortable that my life wasn't ever going to be the way I remember it before cancer again? I did so by practicing the art of surrendering.

I refer to it as the "art of surrendering" because it truly is an art, and like art, it requires some practice. What does it mean to surrender, and whom are you surrendering to?

Most people think that surrendering in your life means to give up. They assume you just leave your fate to the universe or your personal higher power, but that is not at all true. True surrendering means that you recognize there are things in your life you can control and things you can't, and then you relinquish the things you can't control over to a higher power. By doing that, you free yourself from the fear and worry that surrounds the uncontrollable variables in life.

You might be thinking right now, *but I am not religious*. That's okay! When I refer to a higher power, I am not talking about God; this isn't a religious-based practice at all. That's the beauty of it – anyone can do it. Your higher power can be anything. It can be God, but it can also be something else significant to you. It's a personal decision. I refer to my higher power as "the universe," and that is how you will hear me to refer to it in this book. For me, "the universe" encompasses the powers and energy in this world that go beyond my human understanding of things. I always felt the universe guide me in some way throughout my life. Even when bad things happened, I was able to call on my past life experiences and remember the universe had a plan bigger than what I could comprehend. I remind myself that getting where I wanted to go in life wasn't always going to look like I thought it would. I am only human and don't know the right answers all the time. Reminding myself of this helps me avoid worry or question. That is surrender.

What happens when you don't surrender, and you try to control everything in your life? For example, what happened when I was staring at photos and trying to get back to life exactly as it was before cancer? I was in severe emotional pain. I was desperately trying to control things I had no control over. Doing that caused me deep-rooted depression and anxiety. It hurt so badly that eventually, my body, mind, and soul just shut off, and I became numb. I was going through life like a zombie. I couldn't feel joy. I felt like I was having an out of body experience, watching my life as if it was a movie on a screen. I wasn't engaged. I lost my enthusiasm for life, and the things that used to bring me joy felt like chores. I didn't want to work. I didn't want to be around my friends. I just wanted to become invisible.

I can remember the day I surrendered fully. As usual, I woke up with the dread of facing another day, not knowing who I was or how to fit into my life. It was an especially painful day. I couldn't tell you why but looking back, I think I was just at my limit. I remember taking a shower and feeling so weak that I decided just to lay myself in the bathtub and let the water from the showerhead hit my body. I was so desperate to feel anything other than pain and depression. As I let the water run over me, I listened to a meditative chant that reads: "Ek Ong Kar Sat Gur Prasad, Sat Gur Prasad Ek Ong Kar."

The translation is:

God and We are One.
I know this by the Grace of the True Guru.
I know this by the Grace of the True Guru.
God and We are One.

I learned about this mantra years prior in a meditation class, where I learned that these sacred words are believed to stop anything negative and remove all obstacles. It is said that after chanting this mantra, anything you say will be amplified. I was desperate. As I was lying in the tub, chanting the mantra, I gave myself to the universe. I told the universe that I was suffering trying to navigate life on my own and that I knew better. I knew that I couldn't get myself out of this pain and agony and that I needed guidance and hand-holding. I asked the universe to show me the way, and I promised I would open my mind to seeing the path, promising that I wouldn't question it, even if it didn't appear the way I thought it should. I begged the universe to allow me to feel something; I didn't want to be numb anymore.

I got out of the shower, laid on my bed, and immediately it started to happen. I started to cry. Since the day I was diagnosed, I barely cried. I wanted to, but I couldn't. That day, the tears rolled down my face in streams. This went on for hours. It felt as if the universe was pulling the pain from inside me out through my eyes. I went back and forth between sleeping and crying for six straight hours.

From that day forward, things seemed different. I didn't feel as alone. I had faith that there was a bigger plan for me and that every step of the way, if I was in tune, I knew the universe was right next to me.

Besides the obvious relief of the depression and anxiety that surrendering brought, what other gifts has it given me? It has allowed me to feel gratitude. Instead of constantly walking into a wall hoping for it to become a door, I accepted that my life is different, and I am grateful for the new normal. I even learned to feel gratitude for my struggles, as my struggles are opportunities for major growth in my life.

When constructing our new normal, there must include a level of surrender. We can plot, plan, and know what we want, but to be human is to admit that we might not know the best path to get there. You will encounter obstacles, and when you do, you have a choice to make. Do you want to push, fight, and try to control everything, which in turn causes pain and suffering, or do you want to surrender and acknowledge that things happen for a reason, one that you may not understand but will become clear when the time is right?

I can tell you that surrendering is the way to go. You can start right now by identifying your personal higher power and connecting to it. You can connect through prayer, meditation, journaling, conversation, or however you see fit. I go back and forth in my methods of connection depending on what I feel and my needs at the time. One of the ways I stay connected is through the serenity prayer:

God, grant me the serenity
to accept the things I cannot change,
the courage to change the things I can,
and the wisdom to know the difference.

There's that word "God" again. Again, if you aren't religious, just swap it out with a word you are more comfortable with. (Although I consider myself spiritual, I don't consider myself religious. When I recite this prayer, I sometimes swap out "God" for "universe" or "spirit," and sometimes I use "God." Whatever word you want to use is between you and your higher power.)

When defining and accepting our new normal, it is vitally important to accept the things we can't change, change the things we can, and be darn smart enough to know the difference between the two. The things you can change are what you are going to take action on and what you committed to in your letter. In my life, these things show up as eating well, working out, setting boundaries, etc. Examples of things I can't control in my life are others' reactions to my boundaries (for that matter what anyone else does period). And even though I will do what I can to take care of me, I may be able to influence, but I cannot fully control cancer reoccurring. The things you can't change should be released; let them go. Give them up to your higher power. Use the time you would normally use to stress and to try control outcomes to do something more positive with your time. Life is too short to stress over the things you have no control over anyway.

The art of surrender is a step that can't be ignored in this process. We cannot control the fact that cancer came barreling into our lives and changed them forever. We cannot control that our lives will never go back to the normal we once knew. We can, however, accept that we can't control it and put our efforts into making the new normal something we are excited about and proud of and then working hard to make the "new normal" simply "normal."

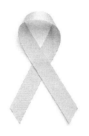

Chapter 7:
Unload Your Burdens

"'No' is a complete sentence."
– Annie Lamott

7

After my experience of surrendering the things I couldn't control to the universe, I felt an overwhelming urge to purge things out of my life that felt heavy and held me down. I realized if I was going to have a "new normal," I had to unload the burdens and the toxins of the "old normal."

One of the first things I did was tear my closet apart. I hoarded so many things in that closet that I mistakenly thought were motivation for me to get back to my old self, but in actuality, were only torturing me. I started by giving away the many pairs of jeans that were too small, relieving myself of the burden of having to fit into them again. Next were shirts that didn't flatter my post-mastectomy breasts. Then I parted with the outfits that had certain memories attached to them, such as the outfit I wore the day before I found out I had cancer – the last day of my old life.

Bathing suits were next, and last but not least, I finally packed up all my bras. I cried during this process.

At many points, especially when I was done, I noticed that I was especially irritable and short-tempered with those around me. I was sad and angry simultaneously. I wasn't just letting go of things; I was packing up memories. In getting rid of these items, I was also terrified I was getting rid of parts of me.

After the initial process of sitting with my emotions, I realized that the items I chose to remove from my closet had nothing to do with removing who I am. I chose to look at it differently. Instead of cancer winning and having to get rid of the old me, making space in my closet was a metaphor for making room in my life. I was making room for the new me. I was allowing space for new clothes, new memories, and happier times. Now, when I walk in my closet in the morning, I feel joy in picking something to wear and not dread, as I am not staring at all the clothes that no longer fit me and probably never would again.

After making it through that experience, I felt like 1,000 pounds were lifted from my chest (no pun intended), and I decided it was time to tackle the next burden weighing me down. I hired a photographer and had new photos taken. It was hard to get in front of the lens with a body I was unsure of and many more scars than I care to admit, but I did it. I continue to have photos taken of me every time I have surgery or something big changes. I no longer want to look at old photos and feel sad; instead, I want to look at current photos and see someone strong and kickass. As a photographer who has photographed many women over my career, I can tell you from both sides of the lens that this experience is incredibly life-changing and powerful. It's one I highly recommend to every woman, especially breast cancer survivors. The experience allowed me to be in my body. I was able to express my inner femininity as well as show my scars and my body as something beautiful and imperfectly perfect. For the first time, in a long time I felt brave, powerful, and damn sexy.

Strong Is the New Sexy

To become someone stronger and be kickass, I knew I had to get back to working out so I could also feel strong. Before cancer, I was a gym rat, and I missed the workouts that I gave my body and my mind. I wasn't sure I wanted to go back to old routines since that would likely bring up comparing myself once again to the old me. Instead, I tried something out of my comfort zone and went to a Muay Thai class (Thai kickboxing). It was love at first punch.

I quickly became obsessed with Muay Thai and wanted to get good at it. It was a struggle at first because I had terrible bone and joint pain from the Lupron shots I was on that suppressed my ovaries. For the first handful of classes, I remember feeling like I wanted to break down and cry right on the mats because every time someone kicked me, it reverberated through every bone in my body, but I didn't give up. Instead, I only pushed harder. To get better at Muay Thai meant trying to lose the post-surgery, post-medical menopause weight I put on. Plus, I had to figure out how to ease the joint pain (I was this close to stopping the Lupron shots, that's how painful it was.) *How am I going to accomplish this?* I wondered.

I saw an integrative practitioner who ran a slew of blood, hair, and urine tests. She put me on a healthier eating plan and on supplements that almost immediately eased my bone pain. I lost about ten pounds over the next few months. Not only did my Muay Thai get better, but my endurance, confidence, and overall wellbeing did also.

As my confidence and the physical side of my life improved, it became clear that the emotional and spiritual aspects of my life were not in alignment. I knew this because I could feel it in the core of my being. There were times when I was around people, or I made life decisions, and my body had internal alarms going off. These alarms showed up in a few different ways. Sometimes it was anger; sometimes, it was an uncontrollable reflex, like sweating or a pit in my stomach. Often, I felt adrenaline rushes or hot flashes that, at first, I contributed to my medication. However, I later realized that it wasn't a coincidence that they would occur at times when I wasn't listening to my intuition. My fuse was certainly shorter, and my bullshit meter was on high alert at all times.

I came to terms that I was a different person, and that new person had different boundaries and needs from relationships and myself. This led me to question everything I thought I knew to be true in my life. This was a deep, soul-searching effort, and one that was extremely painful at times.

Setting Boundaries

I worked on getting curious about all of my beliefs – beliefs about religion, parenting, money, work, marriage, and politics. You name it, I questioned it! While exploring all of my beliefs, I also paid very close attention to where the resistance was in my life and how it made me feel. After a lot of questioning, journaling, hindsight, and therapy, the area I found needed the most work on was in relationships and boundaries. In my work, I discovered that I was a people-pleaser with terrible boundary-setting skills. I was often afraid to speak my mind and held feelings in, possibly to the detriment of my health. I became highly aware of the mind/body connection and how all of the things I was doing in my life over the years that I perceived as "good" and "peacemaking," were hurting me emotionally, spiritually, and in turn, physically.

I learned that when I felt all the terrible feelings that came along with being out of alignment, it was my body and mind begging me to take care of it, asking me to put up a boundary or say no to something I didn't want to do. These feelings were more intense than I ever remember them. It was my intuition guiding me, and it wasn't going to take no for an answer any longer.

Not having boundaries, not speaking your truths, and not knowing how to say no are bad for your health – period. It's not to say that every relationship you are in will be changed post-cancer, but you will know the ones that need to be! Pay attention to the signs your body gives you. Your body knows when it is in the presence of a toxic person or you participate in toxic behavior.

I embraced the principle that if something is not a *hell* yes, it's a no. That applied to so many things in my life. It applies to work and social events, favors people ask of me, and even small things like food or shopping. If I feel something isn't in alignment, I decline it. Why waste time, money, or calories on something you are feeling meh about. Those are our most precious resources, and we should treat them as such. On top of that, I stopped apologizing for not wanting to do something or be around someone. I am not heartless, but I am protective and selective of myself. I was nervous about setting boundaries at first. It certainly took practice! Here's the thing that I didn't know then that I do now. When it is right, it actually feels good to say no. It's empowering, comforting, and genuine. I was such a chronic people pleaser that I was terrified setting boundaries would ruin my relationships. The truth is, it's only made them stronger.

Toxic People

One of the types of people I am careful not to be around is advice-givers. You know who I am talking about; we all have them in our lives. Advice-givers show up in your emails and texts with links to articles titled something like, "Frozen Lemons More Powerful Than Chemotherapy?" or "Hair Dye Associated with Elevated Breast Cancer Rates." In my experience, there is an anxiety that comes with cancer. It doesn't necessarily have to do with dying or being sick, but it has to do with a concern about how I got here. There are many nights when I lied awake in bed and asked myself, *how did I get here?* The thoughts were terrifying. Technically, right now, I don't have cancer, and chemotherapy made sure that any cells that may have escaped are being killed so that I reduce my risk of reoccurrence. So, when people say to me that I should do "this" or I should do "that," it makes me feel like they believe that I did something to cause this cancer in my body.

The truth is, every time I pick up a fork to eat something, I am concerned that I am poisoning my body. Every time I pop a pill in my mouth or have a CAT scan,

I worry. Here's the reality: I don't know anything about medicine. I'm not a doctor, a nurse, or anything even remotely close to either. All of a sudden, I'm thrown into a situation where I'm put in front of a doctor, and she's giving me options for treatment, and I have decisions to make for the rest of my life. It's fucking terrifying. So, when people drop comments or give their opinions on how I should handle my treatment or my post-cancer life, or how you should handle yours, you can kindly let them know you don't need their opinion. Cancer is so individual; it's so unbelievably personal. As cancer patients, we are trying to make the best decisions that we can for ourselves, and we don't know if our decisions are right or wrong, but they are ours to make. So, feel free to say, "thank you, but no thank you," to the advice-givers.

Because these people might mean well, you might find it hard to let them know that what they are doing is hurting you. They might mean well, but in a sense, they are shaming you – shaming you for living your life the way you choose. Nothing gives advice-givers the right to do that, even if they are well-intentioned. You don't have to explain yourself, your choices, or your actions to anyone. When you find that someone you love is an advice-giver, boundaries must be erected, and you can do it lovingly.

You can have a conversation about it, thanking them for being concerned and then letting them know that you have done your research, and you and your doctor are making the best choices for you. Also, it is okay to say, "when you bring me these articles, it actually causes me stress, so if you could please not share them, it would be the best thing you can do for my health and myself." Anyone who loves you will understand, and anyone who doesn't – well, they will eventually disappear.

In times like these, people say you find out who your friends truly are, and they are right! There will be people who drop out of your life. At times, it will feel confusing and difficult, but trust me, if these people can't hang during this time in your life, you will soon discover you are better off without them anyway.

The Theory of Moderation

Cancer is the perfect reason to acknowledge who the toxic people in your life are and clean house. In fact, cancer is the perfect reason to clean up any toxins in your life that don't suit you anymore. When I was diagnosed, I was quickly inundated with information about things I should remove from my life (mostly from the advice-givers). This list included foods, alcohol, clothing, cleaning supplies, beauty products, and more. I refuse to tell you what you should clean up in your life (ugh – that word *should* – it's so dangerous). It's not up to me or anyone else. However, what I will tell you is my theory of moderation.

I changed a lot in my life. I stick to organic food, eat more greens; I take my vitamins and supplements. I hope this, and other changes I made lead to a longer, healthier life, but let me tell you that I'll be damned if I am going to live the rest of my life without pizza, a brownie, or ice cream. I like to color my hair, and this girl needs a good manicure, sometimes even with – gasp – gel polish. As I mentioned before, my theory is that I am always riding a line between doing the healthiest thing I can and living by the motto #YOLO (you only live once). I can't tell you where that line is for you, and neither can anyone else. I can tell you that exploring what living in moderation means to you will help you unload your burdens and accomplish this critical step in your post-cancer life. It is important for you to get clear on your personal post cancer life choices, so the things you do choose to do (like eat that brownie) can be done with joy and happiness because that is the real prescription for good health and long life.

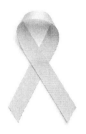

Chapter 8:
The Art of Self-Care

"I have come to believe that caring
for myself is not self-indulgent.
Caring for myself is an act of survival."
— Audre Lorde

8

Now that you worked on cleaning up the toxins in your life, it's time to dig deeper into self-care. Typically, self-care is associated with activities such as hot baths and massages. Those things are great – in fact, I highly recommend them – but that is not the type of self-care I am talking about.

Self-care after cancer involves a deeper level of listening to your body and being in touch with your mind, soul, and your needs more than you have ever imagined before. That often leads to putting yourself first. Chances are if you have responsibilities for other people (for example, if you are married and/or have kids), you have never truly practiced self-care at this level. You are accustomed to taking care of everyone else and ignoring your own needs, or at least putting them on the back burner.

When you start practicing this new depth of self-care, which often involves putting yourself first, your ego is going to step in and tell you that you are being selfish. This is okay and normal. Be aware of it happening and do the best you can to shut it down. I am tempted to say, "it's okay to be selfish." However, the reality is that taking care of yourself isn't selfish. In fact, it's the best gift you can give yourself and those around you. Taking care of you allows you to be happier, healthier, and more present. Remember the instructions on the airplane? Place the oxygen mask over your face before you assist others. That mask is a metaphor for your self-care going forward.

Before I had cancer, I was a ball of energy. I didn't even know we owned a couch – forget actually sitting on it. I was always on the go, and I didn't find that I needed much rest. Then came surgery and chemotherapy; my couch and my bottom got well acquainted.

It was easy to rest post-surgery and during treatment. It was expected that I would need downtime and healing. Once I was done with treatment, I desperately wanted to feel normal and go back to my energetic way of life, so I pushed myself. I remember one particular day; I was in the grocery store with my husband. It was the afternoon, and I already had a pretty full day. We made it to the third or fourth aisle when I just burst into tears. The tears came out of nowhere, and he looked at me panicked. I explained to him that my body was shutting down, and I needed to leave now. He quickly grabbed the cart from my hands, checked out, and got me home.

I had never experienced a shut down like that. It was as if my body was being shut off from the inside, and I couldn't stop it. It was scary and honestly a bit depressing. I was so frustrated that I couldn't even pick a few things up at the store without feeling complete exhaustion. I was done with treatment, so why didn't I just feel normal? I was mad at cancer, mad at my body, and mad at everything.

Through my anger and frustration, I learned a major lesson about rest. I had to learn how to listen to my body's cues and give in to rest when I need it. Sometimes that meant canceling an appointment or asking someone else to carpool. This was not easy for me to do, but I have made it a habit to prioritize rest.

When I successfully make it a priority, I don't experience the shutdowns. In fact, when I rest, everything is easier. Looking back, it took a good twelve to eighteen months to start feeling more myself after chemotherapy. In that time, I mastered the art of the ten-minute power nap and indulge in them regularly without guilt. I no longer "plow through" when I am tired. When making plans, I make sure that I plan accordingly and don't overdo it.

Allowing yourself rest and setting yourself up for success is not only a fierce form of self-care but also of self-love. When I chose to look at it that way, it became much more desirable. Instead of feeling defeated when I ended up on the couch, I feel rewarded.

How did I know when I needed rest? I learned by practicing another form of self-care, namely listening to my intuition. I am a firm believer that the intuition is the strongest muscle in a woman's body and that we should always listen to it. It sounds simple, but we love to complicate it. As women, we shut down our intuition and often allow logic and ego to win. Post-cancer life is the time to strengthen your intuition muscle and pay close attention to what it has to say.

Getting in Touch with Your Intuition

Your intuition is truly the key to your health and wellbeing. When you and your intuition are on the same page, your needs become clear as day. How do you get on the same page? I believe it happens the same way most relationships grow – communication!

When my gut starts acting up and sending me signals that there is a need I am not meeting, I ask it what it's trying to tell me. You don't have to have this conversation out loud and risk people thinking you have an invisible best friend (although that sort of is what your intuition is); this conversation can be had internally. It can come in the form of meditation or something more formal, or it can show up as a quick internal dialogue. That is usually how I work.

If I feel something off in my body, such as a pit in my stomach or an overwhelming feeling to do something or eat something, I stop and ask my body, "What are you trying to tell me? What do you need right now?"

It takes some practice, but the more you do it, the more you will be laser-focused on what you and your body need in the moment to feel your best. (Don't worry – if your invisible best friend is as cool as mine, she doesn't only recommend kale and exercise. She also thinks highly of Netflix, pizza, and red wine!)

The best thing about your intuition (a.k.a. your invisible best friend) is that she goes with you everywhere and she always has your back. This comes in handy when you need a wing woman in life. After I had my implant exchange (from expanders to implants), I was unhappy with how my chest looked. I mentioned it to my plastic surgeon on multiple occasions, but he kept blowing me off. I left his office in tears on more than one occasion.

The last time I saw him, I mentioned again that I was unhappy and asked him if there was anything he could do. His response to me was, "I've seen worse; be happy you are alive!"

When he left the room, my invisible best friend came to life. I knew she was awakened when my stomach was filled with knots. I closed my eyes and asked, "Intuition, what do I do about this?"

My intuition answered, and she told me to be my own advocate. I knew what I had to do. I quickly got dressed and marched myself to the front desk and immediately asked for a transfer of care to a different surgeon.

Wow, did that feel good! I was relieved that I never had to see that insensitive jerk again, but more importantly, I took my power back. I was my own advocate, and I took my power back.

When I finally did see the new surgeon, he took one look at me and said, "Oh no, this is all wrong and not acceptable." I felt validated; I felt strong and proud that I stood up for myself. That experience changed me. It validated me to trust my gut more than ever. It strengthened my relationship with my intuition and now I know I need to trust her implicitly and consider her opinion alongside the others I trust with my care, no matter what their credentials.

Having your intuition on your side also helps manage stress and helps in healing the mind/body connection. Managing stress is critical all the time, but especially post-cancer. Unmanaged stress often manifests in physical symptoms, such as headaches, high blood pressure, stomachaches, and random joint and body pain. Stress can also lead to emotional problems, such as depression, panic attacks, or other forms of emotional distress. In addition to stress, storing trauma in your body can also lead to health issues and further disease. Allow me to break down the word disease for you. It has a different meaning when I present it this way: Dis-ease. Disease is caused by a dis-ease in the body. There's an expression I love that reminds me of this: "the issues are in the tissues."

The issues are in the tissues doesn't just refer to harboring stress, but also to storing any trauma you've experienced throughout your life in the cells of your body. That is how the mind/body connection works. I'm sure you have heard of someone going through a difficult time and suffering from high blood pressure or an ulcer because of it. That is a perfect example of illness caused by internal factors. Now that you are aware of this connection and how it may affect your health, you see why it is vital to not only listen to your intuition but to work through the emotions of the traumas of your life so you can free yourself from the burdens and disease they cause. There are many different ways to heal your past traumas. Modalities such as therapy, hypnosis, and healing energy are just a few examples of the innumerable options out there for deep healing. The method that suits you is a personal decision. I encourage you to keep an open mind and explore the options that call to you. Surrender and listen to your intuition for guidance. Above all else, love yourself and know you are worth the work.

The Practice of Self-Love

Part of self-care is also radical self-love. I use the word "radical" because that is what we need – not some self-love, not self-love most of the time, but the deepest love you can feel. Radical self-love isn't egotistical or selfish. Rather, it's about loving and respecting yourself so deeply that you will do what it takes to live in alignment with what you know you need to be well in your mind, body, and spirit. It's about being so in tune with your spirit that when your spirit tells you what you need, you listen and then act on that knowledge. When your spirit says, "I don't need this right now," radical self-love gives you the strength to make the necessary changes in your life.

Radical self-love is an acceptance of self: the good, the bad, and the ugly.

Cancer is a lonely disease, and I've realized that to survive it, I need to have my back. The only person you are going to be with to the end is you, and radical self-love empowers us to show up for ourselves, standing up for ourselves so that we are fortified for the journey ahead. Radical self-love empowers us because we won't let fear be in the driver's seat anymore. We take our power back and make decisions from a place of strength and love. It's about saying *no* in order to protect our boundaries and make no apologies for that. It's about speaking our minds when we know something isn't right and removing ourselves from toxic people and environments so that we can truly live in alignment with who we are.

Women aren't taught to do this. Instead, we are taught to put everybody else first. I've been good at helping everyone else, but I've finally realized that I need to help myself, and I need to do it now. I am not going to neglect myself to adjust to others, and I am not going to be a people-pleaser. I am going to please myself and do what I know is right for me and my life, because that makes me more peaceful and in turn everything around me more peaceful as well.

The truth is, practicing radical self-love and having the utmost respect for ourselves could save our lives. It helps us make quality decisions about what we eat, do, and let into our lives and bodies. I realize that when I lived out of alignment, it killed my health, motivation, and energy. When I turn my head and shut down my feelings, I suffer. I've suppressed many emotions for so long, and I don't want to do that anymore; that causes cancer. Instead, I choose to take my power back and love myself so fiercely that this love ripples out into my family, my community, and each corner of my life.

I want to change your mind set about the stigma around self-care. Self-care isn't selfish; in fact, I believe it is mandatory to be the healthy person you are meant to be. Health goes way beyond just not having cancer. Remember the oxygen mask analogy? Put your mask on before you help anyone else. You can only take care of others if you yourself are taken care of. Because you are the only one who can hear your gut and physically feel your needs, no one has the potential to take care of you like you do. Self-care is incredibly powerful preventative medicine for all health issues in your life mentally, physically, and spiritually. And the lists of side effects are all good ones. Now that's a pill I am ready to swallow.

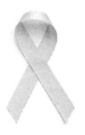

Chapter 9:
Train Your Brain

*"If you don't like something, change it.
If you can't change it, change your attitude."
— Maya Angelou*

9

In 2005, the National Science Foundation published an article summarizing research on human thoughts per day. It was found that the average person has about 12,000 to 60,000 thoughts per day. Of those thousands of thoughts, eighty percent were negative, and ninety-five percent were the same repetitive thoughts as the day before. This proves that one of the tendencies of the mind is to focus on the negative and "play the same songs" over and over again.

There was an additional study (Leahy, 2005, Study of Cornell University) in which scientists found that eighty-five percent of what we worry about never happens. The conclusion is that ninety-seven percent of our worries are baseless and result from an unfounded pessimistic perception. (https://tlexinstitute.com/how-to-effortlessly-have-more-positive-thoughts/)

These statistics are seemingly based on an average person on an average day. What happens when you add cancer into the mix? A dose of fear here, a dab of PTSD there, and it can lead to a recipe for disaster!

In the words of Eckhart Tolle, "The primary cause of unhappiness is never the situation, but the thoughts about it. Be aware of the thoughts you are thinking." My goal for this chapter is to help you identify those thoughts and to give you some tools to combat them.

Cancer and PTSD

Chances are, if you had cancer, you suffer from some level of Post-Traumatic Stress Disorder, also known as PTSD. I always say that breast cancer is as much of a disease of the mind as it is of the breast. The mere thought of cancer coming back can haunt you every single day. Every pain, cough, or change in your body makes your mind immediately question if you have cancer again.

Right around the first anniversary of my mastectomy, I had a routine oncologist appointment. A few days before my appointment, I was in the shower when I felt a lump in my breast. I went to my husband and asked him what he thought it was and immediately had a flashback from the first time I felt a lump. That didn't help my nerves. I showed my oncologist the lump, and she said it was definitely concerning, and she wanted to take a look at it.

"You need to have a sonogram today," she said.

My doctor assured me that when I had my sonogram, the radiologist would talk to me as it was happening, so I wouldn't have to wait and worry. That day, I sat in the cancer center and waited for two hours when they came in to tell me that I needed to come back in another two hours. The waiting only adds to the PTSD and negative thoughts. Time is often our biggest commodity, but also our worst enemy.

The sonogram was emotional for me. My mind kept bringing me back to the last sonogram I had – the one in which I was diagnosed with cancer. It was exactly a year later, and all of a sudden it was happening again. It all felt strangely familiar, as if history was repeating itself, which did not calm my nerves.

Contrary to what I was promised, the radiologist didn't say anything to me during the sonogram. I just kept looking at the screen thinking, *maybe I will recognize if I have cancer or not.*

She remained silent as she worked. The silence was deafening. A few minutes later, she finally announced, "Okay, cover yourself up. I just want to go get the doctor."

When I heard that, I immediately panicked and thought, *Shit, I have cancer again.* She left the room, which meant she left me alone – well, not entirely alone. I was with my thoughts, which were quickly spiraling out of control. It was the longest seven minutes of my life.

I immediately started planning. *This is who I'm going to tell; this is who I'm not going to tell. My daughter is having her bat mitzvah soon, so I'm going to wait until after the bat mitzvah to tell everyone. Where do I want to go before I die? I need to write my children letters. I need them to know how much I love them.* I planned the rest of my life in those seven minutes. Then, the doctor came in and did the sonogram herself.

"It's nothing to worry about," she said nonchalantly. "We think it's a cyst. It's very common when you have a mastectomy that you get oil-filled cysts, and we'll look at it again in three months, just to be sure."

"Aren't you going to biopsy it to check that it's not cancer?" I asked.

"It's really not necessary," she said. "It doesn't fit the qualifications for cancer."

I was so relieved, and at the same time, I was angry. I felt both angry and fortunate that I was reminded in those seven minutes how fragile life is. It was like the universe was giving me a refresher course: *you have a good life right now. You might be struggling with certain things; you may not be feeling great, but you still have opportunities to do things in your life that you want to do. Don't get complacent.*

There are many moments like this post-cancer. You never go into doctors' appointments like you used to, even if they are routine. We need to stay on top of our health. We get MRIs, PET scans, colonoscopies, etc. The nerves, fears, and thoughts that come along with that are exhausting. "Scanxiety" is a real thing; it can all be very overwhelming.

It can also be overwhelming when you *don't* have health issues, just waiting for the other shoe to drop. I don't know about you, but I think about cancer every single day in one way, shape, or form.

Two years after I finished treatment, a close family member of mine was diagnosed with cancer. I was there every step of the way to support him through his extremely difficult journey. The emotions and thoughts I experienced during that time were intense. There were times when he was getting a needle, and I could feel it in my veins. My cancer was difficult, but his cancer just threw me over the edge. That was when I realized that my PTSD was real, and I couldn't ignore it anymore.

I'm not a doctor, and certainly, I don't specialize in PTSD treatment, but I can speak about it from my point of view. I am not sure that PTSD is ever one-hundred percent curable, but I do know that I found ways that truly help me when I have dark thoughts and difficult days.

Training Your Brain

Your brain is a muscle, and just like any other muscle in your body, it can be trained. Imagine yourself in the gym doing bicep curls. You don't walk out of the gym with buff arms after one visit; it takes many visits and sometimes even some struggle and pain to get the desired results. Training your brain works the same way; it takes practice and fortitude.

This is how I work on training my brain. My first and most important tip is to simply ask yourself if what you are thinking and/or feeling is real and the truth. Sometimes it is, but most often, it isn't! Remember, of those thousands of thoughts we think every day, eighty percent are negative, and ninety-five percent are exactly the same repetitive thoughts as the day before. Odds are, the negative thoughts you think are *not* real and don't deserve your attention. Asking myself whether or not my thought is real, helps me figure out where I stand pretty quickly.

For me, I find fear is the biggest culprit. It's the emotion and thought that pops up the most, and it's also the biggest liar. It puts untrue thoughts in my head, such as, "It's only a matter of time before your cancer comes back." This thought is solely based on fear, not on fact. Fear is not a black and white emotion; there are levels of grey in fear. For example, your fear of cancer returning is, of course, legit; however, it is not your current reality. We can only deal with what is in front of us today. This is a practice in surrender once again. As I write this chapter, ironically, we are in the midst of the coronavirus pandemic. Left and right things are being shut down; the stock market is crashing, plus my kids are home and out of school for an undetermined amount of time.

This morning, I woke up feeling particularly anxious. There are legitimate reasons to be fearful right now. Our health is at risk, people are losing their jobs and we aren't sure when it is going to come to an end. Life is very uncertain right now. It's easy to get swallowed up by this fear. Because this fear is legitimate, it can quickly lead to a downward spiral of dark thoughts. Personally, I start wondering if my business is going to make it, how I will pay my bills, and what happens if one of my family members falls ill.

This is a good example of fear not being black or white. Because I know that fear can be legitimate and at the same time not real, I had to stop and take a big breath this morning. I asked myself, *is your fear real?* The answer was yes *and* no. I knew that I had reasons to feel fear, but I also had to limit it and check in with reality. The reality is that in this moment, my family is healthy. I have a roof over my head and plenty of food (and toilet paper) at home. I built my business once; I will do it again if I have to. I also realize that when I check in with myself, I don't have control over what happens in the world. I repeat the serenity prayer a few times, and I remember that I can only control what I can – which is my reaction to what happens.

The same is true post-cancer. It's incredibly easy to get caught in the dark, downward spiral of negative thinking. It's much harder to stay positive, but that is what this training is all about. It's not to say you won't have bad days or that you are not entitled to them in the first place. You are entitled to bad days; I have them too, and often, I embrace them. Truthfully, there is nothing as soul-cleansing as a good, messy, heartfelt cry. You can't positive think yourself out of everything; some things are just downright scary. Allow yourself to have those feelings. When I am done having those feelings, and I wipe away the tears, I implement another tactic to help. I turn to gratitude.

Gratitude

Gratitude is a quick, free, and easy way to improve your mental health. Having and practicing gratitude releases a multitude of toxic emotions and releases dopamine and serotonin in our brain. Dopamine and serotonin are the two neurotransmitters that enhance our moods. In layman's terms, gratitude makes us happy. Feeling gratitude attracts more gratitude. It's a win-win. Practicing gratitude is so easy.

Here are a few ways I do it:

- Write down 3 – 5 things you are thankful for every night before going to bed.
- Say thank you. This can be to anyone you feel deserves it. A family member, doctor, friend, or stranger. Although being thankful is an act, gratitude is the feeling that will accompany it.
- Give a compliment. This is one of the most powerful ways of sharing love and happiness.
- Practice random acts of kindness. Pay for someone's coffee, send someone flowers, mail a letter to someone special, the options are endless.
- Find things to be thankful for in the hardest parts of your life. This means finding gratitude in your struggle and fears. Finding gratitude helps remove the power from the darkness.

There are so many ways to practice gratitude. It doesn't matter how you do it; it only matters that you do it. Gratitude is a form of love. As time goes on, you will find the more you give, the more you attract gratitude. The exchange of positive energy that gratitude cultivates not only feels good, but it also heals.

When all else fails, and the fear and negativity seem overwhelming, I call on the big guns. I actively pump myself up. I ask myself, *do you want to be a worrier or a warrior?* The answer is always warrior. We envision warriors as strong, bulletproof figures, always ready for battle, and who are fearless to the bone, but I don't believe that to be true. I think true warriors are fearless, but to me, fearless doesn't mean operating without fear. Instead, it means moving forward despite of fear. Adversity, fear, and worry are always going to pop up in our lives. We can't control those, but we can control how we think and react to them. This is so powerful because it's the story we create that allows for the experience.

So, let me ask you, what do you want to be? I know your answer is a *warrior* – because you already are one. The only way to be a warrior over a worrier is to work on your brain like a muscle. Keep repeating the same fear-fighting, negative-thought-crushing, and PTSD-destroying behaviors over and over. Use my tips, or find something that works for you, and practice it over and over again and train that brain!

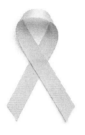

Chapter 10:
Own Your Power

*"Acceptance of what has happened
is the first step to overcoming the consequences
of any misfortune."*
— William James

10

To take steps to put your life back together, there needs to be a healthy acceptance of what you have been through. This acceptance is a process to achieve. It takes time and if I am honest, it can often be painful. There is great beauty on the other side of the pain. Acceptance instills a sense of power in you that is life-changing. Owning that power fuels you to change your life.

The Five Stages of Grief

You may have heard of the five stages of grief, also known as the Kübler-Ross model, created by Elizabeth Kübler-Ross. Kübler-Ross worked with terminally ill patients for years to come up with this model of how people process grief. It was later adapted for other experiences with loss, which I think we all can agree, cancer is.

The five stages of grief are:

- Denial
- Anger
- Bargaining
- Depression
- Acceptance

There is no hard and fast rule to grief and getting to the point of acceptance. The process takes a different amount of time for everyone. It's also not linear. You may find you go back and forth between stages, and you may even skip stages. There's no perfect way to grieve. You need to do it on your timeline, in your way, but you do need to do it. In this chapter, I am going to break down the steps and how they apply to us as breast cancer survivors. Knowing these stages will serve as a roadmap to help you navigate your journey.

Denial

Getting diagnosed with cancer is shocking. You are confused and overwhelmed. You hear what the doctor says, and you understand it, but somehow it feels like a bad dream you are going to wake up from any minute. It's hard to believe. Denial is a natural defense mechanism, numbing you from the intensity of your feelings, which allows you more time to absorb the news. This is a funny stage. I don't quite remember being in denial, but then I think that must be the denial doing its job.

Sometimes even years after my diagnosis, I am still in shock and denial. It's a lot to absorb in a short period of time. If denial still sneaks up on you now and again, know you aren't alone in that.

Anger

There is so much emotion to process in your cancer journey and post-cancer life. It's natural to feel anger after the denial wears off. Anger can be expressed in many ways, and this is often the stage where you ask, "Why me?" or look for something to blame. Anger can often be disguised as other emotion. For example you might find yourself holding on to resentment, feeling frustrated or maybe you are easily irritated. For me, anger and bargaining showed up simultaneously.

Bargaining

Bargaining comes with feeling vulnerable and helpless. This is where you might find yourself asking, "what if" questions. This is also the stage where surrender to a higher power often exists.

For my whole life, I took good care of my body. I always did what I thought was the right thing to do to avoid illness. I worked out, drank green juice, and did yoga. I didn't have a history of cancer in my family, so it wasn't something I worried about. However, that didn't stop me from doing what I could to avoid disease.

When I was diagnosed with cancer, I couldn't help but lay awake at night, questioning what I did to cause it. Did I eat something I shouldn't have? Maybe it was that darn Keto diet or years of toxic nail polish. I started to trace back everything I ever did, every place I had ever been to, and everything I put on or in my body. The week I was diagnosed, I lost seven pounds because I was terrified of eating anything. Everything seemed like poison to me. I tried to eat, and a voice in my head would whisper, "Maybe *this* is what caused your cancer."

My emotions soon went from fear to anger. I was angry with my body. "I took care of you!" I thought, "Why would you turn on me?" I saw my body as my enemy. It was the first time in my life that I realized what somebody on a premature deathbed might feel like. I remember closing my eyes and saying to my body, *my soul isn't done yet. Don't give up on me, because my soul isn't done yet. Why are you turning on me? I'm not ready.*

There is nothing more confusing than trying to live in and love a body that has turned on you. How do you reconcile with the enemy? The truth is that it's so difficult to love your body when it is turning on you, but this is the time your body needs it the most.

Learning to love my body even though it turned against me was a challenge, and it also taught me so much. I used meditation and affirmations I learned to change my vocabulary and thoughts.

When I feel a negative thought come into my head about my body, I try to cut myself off and use an affirmation or mantra such as, "I'm grateful for my body; my body is powerful," or "have patience and grace with yourself."

Doing this stops the thought in its tracks and immediately distracts me from going down a negative road because that road is dark. Negative thoughts perpetuate anger towards my body and cancer. That anger is only going to perpetuate disease in my body, so I need to free myself of that anger. Meditation, positive self-talk, gratitude, and mantras/affirmation are all ways I have been able to lean into the feeling and then let it go, releasing my body of the burden.

When I started chemotherapy, I had an eye-opening revelation about my body. Chemotherapy is quite literally poison. It is an unbelievably insane act for a human to voluntarily hook himself or herself up to poison, week after week. It gets more absurd as time goes on, and you feel worse and worse. On days that I was leveled, nauseous, tired, and just done, I could hear my body asking, *why are you doing this to me? I don't understand. You're putting me in the chair and plugging me into poison. Why are you treating me this way?* The response that came to my mind was, it's what I have to do to get rid of the enemy – and there it was.

That was the exact moment I realized that it wasn't my body that was the enemy; it was the cancer. Instead of this battle being me against my body, I realized it was me and my body against cancer. This perspective is a game-changer. Once you acknowledge your body is actually your teammate in the battle, you can let go of the anger and find gratitude for it. Once you find gratitude, you can take the next step in moving towards owning your power and achieving acceptance.

Depression

There are many opportunities for depression to strike during cancer. Your life is uprooted; you are potentially losing your breasts and/or hair, along with much of your identity. Work is disrupted, relationships are stressed, and you feel like crap. Everything you once knew is different overnight. Depression is not just extreme sadness. It's common to withdraw from life, feel numb, and live in a fog.

Depression looks different and hits at different times for everyone. In my case, depression hit me almost immediately after my treatment was over. I finished treatment on December 27, 2017. I was ready to start the New Year fresh and energized, but that isn't quite what happened.

Three weeks into 2018, I found myself frustrated and lost. I was done with treatment, yet I didn't feel better. I was expecting joy and life, but instead, I felt alone and scared. I started my hormone blocker, Tamoxifen. It gave me hot flashes and kept me awake at night. Everyone in my life kept asking me how happy I was that I was done with treatment and that I was officially a survivor, finally able to get on with life. In public, I put on a happy face and pretended that I was okay and happy, but I was far from okay.

On that January day, I had a photoshoot in the morning. I struggled to get out of bed, but I knew in the back of my mind that if I went, it would be a good distraction. I barely made it through the shoot without falling apart. After the shoot, I drove home, went to my bedroom, crawled into bed, shut off my phone, and just shut down.

That was a memorable day because it was the first time in my life that I ever experienced suicidal thoughts. I couldn't help but think that if I took my own life, I would relieve not only myself but also all of my loved ones from the hell that cancer put us through. Before cancer, I was a happy, fit, joyous, confident woman. In bed that day, I was a fearful, worn down, exhausted excuse for a human. I fought so hard to save my life, and that was how I was expected to live? I didn't want to live that way for another minute.

I am so grateful that along with the suicidal thoughts existed my logic. My logical voice told me I was being ridiculous. There was a war in my mind, but the logical side won. I was able to get out of bed that day and every day after, but it wasn't easy most days.

My depression manifested in numbness and isolation. I stopped seeing most of my friends. I went to work events that I always loved and got such satisfaction out of, and I would feel as if I wasn't there. I couldn't get in touch with any emotions. I wasn't getting joy from activities that previously gave me great joy. I had no interest in doing much; I was numb.

During that time, I didn't know how to explain to anyone in my life how I felt. There was so much pressure to "just be grateful" that I felt stupid and selfish. That was when I decided to seek out the help of a therapist. It was through therapy that I was able to reconnect with my emotions about what I had been through. Those emotions were dark, and it was difficult to face them, but when I did, it was as if a new world was open to me.

Acceptance

Acceptance is the part of the journey where your emotions stabilize. You realize you will have to build a new normal life post-cancer, and you are okay with that. You don't look at having cancer as something good that happened to you, but you are able to find the silver linings. Acceptance doesn't mean you won't have bad days or not experience the other stages of grief, but you know if you do, you will be okay.

Why is getting to a place of acceptance so important? Once you have been touched by cancer, it will always be a part of your life. You are either fighting it, or you have no evidence of disease, but you are still aware that you need to do what you can to prevent a reoccurrence. Acceptance helps you make the changes you need to feel normal again. In fact, nothing in this book will work without acceptance of what we have been through and our challenges ahead. Accepting that you had cancer and that it is part of your story is so powerful. It shifts the power back to you and robs the cancer of it. When you have power, you are capable of anything.

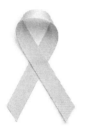

Chapter 11:
Reconnect with
Your Femininity

"Beauty isn't about having a pretty face.
It's about having a pretty mind,
a pretty heart, and a pretty soul."
– Anonymous

11

Breast cancer isn't just an attack on your body and your life; it declares a full-on war on your femininity. Whether you have a lumpectomy, mastectomy, oophorectomy, hysterectomy, lost your hair, were put into menopause, all of the above, or none of the above, just being diagnosed with breast cancer is enough to feel your femininity being threatened. In my case, I was forty-one years old, presumably in the prime of my life. I was in pretty good shape, felt good about my health and my age, and then out of nowhere, my life was drastically altered. In this chapter, I will share my struggles with you about feeling normal in my body and offer some advice on how to reconnect with your femininity.

I struggled with body image issues throughout my life, but ironically, I always loved my breasts. In the moment, choosing to remove my breasts was a no-brainer. I had two large masses in one breast, and who knows what was lingering in the other (turns out I had Lobular

Carcinoma in situ (LCIS) in the other breast. LCIS isn't cancer but being diagnosed with it indicates you have a higher risk of developing breast cancer.). No doubt, it was the right decision. In fact, when I made the decision, I was relieved, not upset. Having an action plan allowed me to feel in control. Instead of counting down to my breasts being removed, I counted down to the days to the cancer being removed.

Femininity Under Attack

When I got dressed the morning of my mastectomy, I was cognizant of what I wanted to wear. I wore a cute pair of ripped jeans, a camouflage T-shirt (battle-ready), and a pair of hot pink Manolo Blahnik high heels that I coincidentally splurged on just a few days before my diagnosis. The nurses and doctors got a good chuckle from the shoes and told me they had never seen anyone wear heels to a mastectomy before, and certainly not hot pink heels. It wasn't just a fashion statement; it was my way of reminding myself that femininity doesn't have to be defined by my breasts or even my body. There are ways I can think and feel feminine, regardless of having a mastectomy. Even after my breasts were removed, I didn't feel sadness; I felt relief. I felt strong and powerful. Then I went through chemotherapy, and even though that knocked me on my ass, I still felt like a soldier plowing through enemy ground. It wasn't until after my implant exchange surgery healed that I started to notice certain feelings change.

Boob envy is a real thing, and I started to feel it more and more. To add salt to the wound, my job requires me to see women in lingerie or unclothed all the time. I greatly miss my nipples and having feeling in my chest. I hate that I don't have cleavage and that finding clothing to flatter my body is so difficult. The boob envy, the sadness, and the feeling of being robbed of femininity didn't occur immediately after my mastectomy. Instead, it was a tidal wave that hit after treatment and reconstruction surgery was over.

After being put on Lupron shots (another attack on femininity), I went to see my OB/GYN for my yearly physical and to discuss removing my ovaries. I sat in the packed waiting room, looking around at all the beautiful pregnant women. They looked young and glowing, and I couldn't help but feel the pit in my stomach that I wasn't like them anymore. I went into that appointment sure that I was going to book my surgery, but the minute the doctor started talking about it, I burst into tears, which surprised both the doctor and me.

"But you are done having kids," my doctor said with a confused look on her face. I didn't expect her to get it. It's not about that. It's about being engaged in yet another attack.

After that appointment, I felt exhausted. I cried. I felt old washed up. I wondered if my best days were behind me. I looked in the mirror and didn't recognize myself. I started to think that the surgeries, treatments, medications, stress, and side effects were finally catching up to me and turning me into someone I didn't want to be. I had to get real with myself. I knew I had to redefine where my femininity came from, internally and externally.

Seeing through a Different Lens

When I was going through chemotherapy, I had the absolute pleasure of photographing a breast cancer survivor who I met online. Her name is Marianne, and she is a three-time cancer survivor. She had a mastectomy and, after complications from reconstruction, decided to go flat. I spent the day with Marianne, listening to her stories of bravery. I watched her step out of her comfort zone and bare it all for my camera. We filmed a video about what sexy meant to her and where she finds it from now that she doesn't have breasts. The experience was incredibly touching and moving. When she left for the day, I was filled with wonder and amazement at her courage and strong feminine energy. I turned to my friend and make-up artist, Diana and said, "Isn't she amazing? I wish I could be like her!"

Diana cocked her head to the side and replied, "Jen, you *are* like her!"

At that moment, I was reminded that we couldn't possibly see ourselves the way other people see us.

When I see other breast cancer survivors, they always seem healthy, whole, beautiful, and strong. Are they seeing *me* that way too?

It was clear that I didn't have it in myself to feel that way, but I did have the ability to pull from how others see me when I can't find it within myself. I tried to change some external things. I bought a new red lipstick. I bought all new lace undies that make me feel girly when I put them on. Hey, if I couldn't wear bras, at least I had that! I tried to dress up more, but it wasn't enough to make physical changes.

I essentially had to change my mind about what femininity is. If it wasn't my breasts or my fertility, what was it? Where did it come from? I sat down with my journal, and I made a list of all the strengths and qualities I found in other women in my life. Things on my list included characteristics such as:

- Determined
- Loving
- Funny
- Caring
- Strong
- Intelligent
- Dedicated
- Trailblazing
- Spicy
- Bold
- Hard-working

The list goes on and on. Right away, I noticed that not one thing on the list had to do with anything physical. All the qualities I adored in other women, that defined who they are, were so much deeper.

I then wrote a list about myself. I first started with what I thought others saw in me, and then I wrote a list of what I wanted to be known for. Again, none of those qualities had anything to do with any physical attributes. If that is the case, that must mean that my femininity can't be taken by removing physical aspects of my body. In fact, I may even argue that cancer amplified all of the qualities that define me as a woman. I am now stronger, more sensitive, and more present and loving. I am certainly spicier and more determined than ever. My femininity is expressed in how I handled the adversity that was thrown at me and how I showed up as a woman. That is what I remind myself of when I feel down or under attack. In redefining my femininity, I focus on who I want to be, how I want to leave my mark in this world, and how I want to show up as a friend, spouse, and mother. I learned how to redefine myself as a woman through changing my standards of what being feminine is, but there is still one area where the physical cannot be escaped, and that's in the bedroom.

Sex and Cancer

Feeling like you are losing your femininity has a ripple effect on many areas of life, including your sex life. Let's be honest; you don't feel super sexy when you're going through chemotherapy and radiation and healing from surgeries. Your body hurts and feels alien. You're exhausted. You may even feel a loss of sexual desire. I don't have nipples or breast sensitivity, which are a great loss in the pleasure of sex. I can't lay on my stomach, and I couldn't even roll on my side for months. Even just pressing up against my husband for a hug felt uncomfortable at times. All of these physical and emotional side effects of cancer take a toll on your sex life.

My body looks different than it did before cancer; I have scars and deformed breasts. I've also gained some weight and lost muscle. I don't feel as confident naked as I used to. There are many women I know whose partners won't look at them after cancer and surgery; I've heard stories of men who even leave their wives. However, it wasn't that way with my husband. He always thought I was beautiful. My hope was always that my husband would look at my scars the way I do, that I can do anything, and I am strong, and he has.

Still, the sex changed. How could it not? I've changed. When you are with someone long enough, there is a sort of familiar dance to sex. You know where you will be touched, or what your partner's next move is; there is a comfort in that. Now, the dance needs to be reworked. It doesn't work as it used to. It hurts, or you don't feel it, or there aren't nipples to touch. There is mourning in that.

I believe that to heal, it's important to be honest. It's important to keep the communication between you and your partner open which allows for a new level of intimacy, physically and emotionally. Don't be afraid to speak up and say when something hurts or isn't pleasurable. Your body has gone through a trauma, and it deserves deep care and mindfulness from both you and your partner. Even more importantly, don't be afraid to speak up when something is pleasurable. What I have found is that when I can experience pleasure in my body, it helps me reconnect with it, and it allows me to feel sexy and feminine.

If your sexual activity has changed or disappeared, there are still ways you and your partner can stay connected. Many nights my husband would give me a massage, and this helped me in so many ways. It helped distract my mind from pain and feel pleasure instead. It allowed us to have intimate contact. Although it wasn't sex, it was something special between just us. It allowed both of us time to understand my body and what felt good – and yes, some nights, the massages led to more intimate things. The point is that the massages, and other things like cuddling, allowed us to take things slowly. We both had to realize that we could never go back to our sex life before cancer; we had to create a new dynamic.

Between reevaluating how to define femininity, working on taking back my sexuality, and owning the qualities that make me who I am as a woman, I feel stronger and more in touch with myself than I have ever felt before. It helped solidify my relationship with myself and helped me grow into a person I am proud to be. I realized that I am actually more feminine than I have ever been. I realized I thought about it all wrong. It might seem that cancer was trying to steal my femininity, but the truth is that by overcoming the challenges placed before me, cancer has actually given me the gift of being even more determined, loving, funny, caring, strong, intelligent, dedicated, trailblazing, spicy, bold, hard-working, and therefore more feminine than I have ever been. By following the tips in this chapter, you too can create a new dynamic and own your fierce femininity.

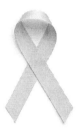

Chapter 12:
Embracing Joy

"When you do things from your soul,
you feel a river moving in you, a joy."
— Rumi

12

"How do you look so beautiful and happy? I don't understand. My life has been overrun with sadness and PTSD. I can't find joy after cancer," a woman recently commented after watching one of my YouTube videos about my cancer journey.

She was in the stage of finishing treatment and putting her life back together. My response to her was something I wish someone said to me.

"I give you permission to feel the sadness *and* have joy. The two conflicting emotions *can* live within you at the same time. So, if that means you need to take a trip, go. If you want to create art, sign up for a class or just buy paint and paper and begin. Watch a movie, take a bath, hang out with your friends, laugh, do whatever it is that brings you joy, make it a priority every single day. If you don't know what brings you joy, make it your mission to discover it. You deserve this." And now, my friend, I say the same thing to you. In this chapter, I will help you find what brings you joy and help you embrace it.

The Benefits of Joy

The woman wrote me back to say that she never thought about the conflicting emotions being present at the same time. If you haven't thought about it that way either, I encourage you to acknowledge that even though you might be sad, angry, tired, or any other emotion, joy is your ally as you rebuild your life. You have permission to feel joy even though you have cancer. You have permission to feel joy even when you struggle, and you have permission to feel joy even when life feels overwhelming, and you feel like you're falling behind.

It is absolutely vital to experience joy in life. Why? Joy changes our brains and our bodies. (https://www.healthline.com/health/affects-of-joy#1) According to healthline.com, we feel joy in our neurotransmitters, which are tiny chemical "messenger" cells that transmit signals between neurons (nerves) and other bodily cells. Those neurotransmitters are responsible for processes and feelings in almost every aspect of the body, from blood flow to digestion.

Feeling more joy also has other benefits, and it:
- Promotes a healthier lifestyle
- Boosts immune system
- Fights stress and pain
- Supports longevity

We feel joy in our bodies because of the release of dopamine and serotonin, two types of neurotransmitters in the brain. Both of these chemicals are heavily associated with happiness. In fact, to prove how powerful joy is, even just by smiling, you can trick your body into feeling joy; it doesn't even have to be based on real emotion! Now that you know there is proof that body and your emotions work in tandem, it may be more enticing to feel more joyful on a daily basis.

Using Joy to Overcome Hard Times

I find joy to be particularly important around meaningful dates, such as anniversaries that can drum up many emotions. The first anniversary of my cancer diagnosis was much harder than I thought it was going to be. I envisioned it to be a celebration. I survived the year and thought it was going to be great, but that was not the case. As the day approached, I got more and more anxious and upset. I got my kids ready to go to a sleepaway camp like I do every year, and there was something about the ritual of this that just leveled me.

I was folding their clothes and thinking, *this time last year I was fine. This time last year, cancer was in my body, and I didn't know. This time last year, my kids were innocent and had no care in the world.*

My husband and I went to drop our kids off at camp, and I felt so anxious that it was difficult to breathe. The more we did things that were similar to the days leading up to my diagnosis, the harder it got.

When the first anniversary finally arrived, I felt as if I had a big, black cloud all around me and didn't know what to do. What do you do with a year that changed your life forever? What I thought would be a celebration turned into a day in which I just wanted to be alone. There were a lot of flashbacks and PTSD. What I ended up doing that day was total self-care. I surrendered and allowed myself just to feel terrible. It was a horrible, emotional, and miserable day.

I learned a lesson that day. I learned that it's probably best to plan ahead for these anniversaries. After making it through my diagnosis anniversary, I knew my mastectomy anniversary was right around the corner. I was going to be ready for it.

My husband looked at me like I was crazy when I told him I wanted to go to Paris in two short weeks for my mastectomy anniversary. I told him I didn't care what the trip cost or how many points we needed – I would do whatever it took because I didn't want to be home on

August second. Instead, I wanted to create new memories for the day and start working on my bucket list (Paris was number one on the list).

It took some arm twisting, but on the first of August, we boarded that plane to Paris! We arrived on the second and spent the next few days there (including my birthday). It was a dream trip. I spent that day shopping, eating, and indulging in Parisian life, without a moment to feel bad for myself. Taking that trip was more than just a distraction; it was a celebration of life. It was all about making a new memory for the day. Now, I can look back on that anniversary and remember it's the anniversary of my first time in Paris. Even now, when I think about that weekend, I feel joy in my whole body.

I realize that hopping on a plane to Paris is extravagant and not always a realistic way to overcome hard times. The moral of the story isn't about Paris. The moral of the story is that it doesn't matter what you do or how you make a new memory, just that you put the effort in to do so. By doing that, you are changing the narrative around these important dates, which allows you to shed depression and anxiety and make room for extreme joy.

What Does Joy Feel Like?

What does joy feel like? How do you know when you are living with the vibrations of joy? One of the ways I use to identify where I am in the emotional range is referring to the Abraham-Hicks emotional guidance scale. The scale represents twenty-two of our most felt emotions. The higher up, the happier and higher the vibration, and the lower on the scale, the less happy and lower the vibration. Vibration is referring to the overall state of being energetically speaking. Your vibration at any given moment is made up of the vibrational frequency from your emotional, physical, and spiritual energy fields. Simply put, the higher your vibration, the better you feel in each of the three pillars of wellness.

To use this scale, all you have to do is identify which emotion you feel at the moment. Once you identify where you are, you have a choice of how to proceed. You can choose to move up the scale (raise your vibration), or down the scale (lower your vibration). As you can see, joy is the highest metric on the scale. Along with joy comes appreciation, empowerment, freedom, and love.

Emotional Scale

1. Joy/appreciation/empowered/freedom/love
2. Passion
3. Enthusiasm/eagerness/happiness
4. Positive expectation/belief
5. Optimism
6. Hopefulness
7. Contentment
8. Boredom
9. Pessimism
10. Frustration/irritation/impatience
11. Overwhelm
12. Disappointment
13. Doubt
14. Worry
15. Blame
16. Discouragement
17. Anger
18. Revenge
19. Hatred/rage
20. Jealousy
21. Insecurity/guilt/unworthiness
22. Fear/grief/depression/despair/powerlessness

– From the book *Ask and It Is Given,* by Esther and Jerry Hicks

So, let's say, for example, I was around a nine or ten on my diagnosis anniversary. I made a choice not to hang in that zone again; it didn't feel good, and I didn't like it. Once a few days passed, I was back at contentment (seven), but looking forward, I knew I was bound to repeat the cycle of moving back down the scale as my mastectomy anniversary approached. Then I had the idea of going to Paris. After that, I was in the five or six range. I told my husband I wanted to go to Paris and once we booked the trip, I was in the three to four range. Immediately after that, I got to two since Paris was so high up on my bucket list and I felt so passionate about going. While in Paris, I was no doubt at a one. Even as I wrote this and thought about that trip, my eyes filled with tears of joy, and my body and mind felt lighter.

Finding Joy in the Every Day

Of course, the Paris example is great, but let's be honest, most days are much more mundane. However, make no mistake, the scale can also be used in your daily life and experiences. Remember, at the beginning of the book, when I said there was a huge difference between being alive and feeling alive? For me, joy involves any activity that helps me feel alive. For example, participating in the Muay Thai class, I mentioned earlier, gives me joy.

The class was a challenge, to say the least. Besides the problems like body pains that I previously mentioned, I also had a hard time holding the pads for my partner because I had lost most of my muscle strength.

During the class, I was out of breath, and I felt like I had cinder blocks on my feet. It sounds awful, and a lot of times it was but believe it or not, I loved it. I felt so much joy in pushing my body. It made me feel *incredibly* alive. Even the moments of pain and difficulty led to extreme gratitude for what my body could do and that I was healthy enough to be there. This was a huge perspective shift for me (a moment of training my brain).

When I struggled to keep up, and everything hurt, I changed my internal dialogue from, "This is hard," "This sucks," and "I can't do this," to "I am so lucky to *get* to do this," and "I am doing it for someone who can't today."

To this day, I still incorporate Muay Thai into my life about three times a week. Without it, I find myself slipping down the scale again and living in zones sixteen to twenty-two, which is not where I want to be.

Another thing that brings me joy is being creative, or as I call it "art therapy." Painting, drawing, writing, and any other type of creating gives me space to think and breathe. It helps me relieve myself of my feelings by getting them out, acknowledging them, and making space for them. It's almost an active meditation for me. In moments of high stress, I find that my art therapy never fails me.

Joy can sometimes sneak up on you without even knowing it. Sadly, three weeks after my mastectomy, my dog of 12 years suddenly passed away. It was gut-wrenching for my family and me. Not that there is any good time for something like that, but this time was particularly raw. We decided not to get a new dog until after my treatment was done. That time came and went, but I still wasn't ready for a new dog. In fact, I was ok without a dog if I am honest. Most of the responsibilities of my previous dog fell on me, and I just didn't need the burden. As time went on, my family was begging me for a dog. I begrudgingly went to a dog adoption event one fateful day in November 2018. The last thing I said to my family before we walked in was, "Don't forget, we are NOT getting a dog."

Next thing I know, we are walking out with the cutest little 6-pound straggly rescue puppy I have ever seen. His name is Tex. When we got Tex, I wasn't in the best mind frame. Cancer was on my mind, a lot. Way more than I wanted it to be. So much so that it started feeling normal just to live life consumed with thoughts. When Tex came along, I worked from home so I could housebreak him and keep him company. The truth is, he was keeping me company. After a few days of puppy cuddles and many walks, I realized I hadn't thought about cancer in days. The thought brought tears to my eyes. I felt free, even if for a brief moment. As a bonus, I felt extreme love and joy from our new family member and still do every day.

In addition to things I do regularly to feel joy, I also make sure I incorporate new experiences in my life. One friend of mine and I made a pact to take one day a month to try something new. It might be trying a new restaurant, rock climbing, floating in a float tank, or doing something completely out of our comfort zone. Not only is it fun to experience something new but doing it with a close friend also brings even more joy.

Besides participating in activities, there are other ways to move your emotions up the scale and vibrate at a higher level. Once you identify where you are in the moment, you can use practices such as meditation and positive thinking to help to raise your vibration. The important thing to know here is that it is best to move up the scale one emotion at a time. As Abraham Hicks says, "Reach for a better feeling thought."

Positive thinking is amazing, but if you plan on positive thinking yourself straight from jealousy to passion, you will be frustrated and disappointed. Instead, take it one step at a time. When you do this, you will see that life around you will start matching your high vibration. The more joy you feel, the more joy you will attract; the more you attract, the better life is. The better life is, the healthier you are. The healthier you are, the more alive you will feel. I could go on. I hope I have helped you see that joy is a key ingredient in life and health. It's the key to a full and vital life. Keep a tally on what brings you joy and then add it to your life every single day. Whether it's a once in a lifetime trip or a walk down the street, find joy in the big and small. Find it in the mundane and exciting. If you can't find it, create it. I promise you, joy is a game-changer.

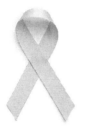

Chapter 13:
Community

*"One of the most important things
you can do on this earth
is to let people know
they are not alone."*
— *Shannon L. Alder*

13

One week before I started chemotherapy, I went out to dinner with a bunch of local couples after back-to-school night. It was September; the new school year was just underway, and everyone was getting back into the swing of real life again – except for me. I was about to embark on eight treatments (sixteen weeks) of chemotherapy.

At the dinner, there was the usual deluge of complaints. "I can't believe we have to get back to real life," "Ugh, I can't believe we have to pack lunches again," or "I hate waking up at seven a.m."

With every complaint, I felt my jealousy grow deeper. All I wanted was the ability to be free to take care of my children, make lunches, drive carpool, and have a life free of cancer. With every bone in my body, I just wanted to go back to normal.

It's funny how cancer changes your perspective. Your biggest problems in life immediately become your smallest problems. The things you hated and took for granted prior, you now wish for in your life. For me, I found that this perspective shift made it difficult for me to be around certain people. It wasn't their fault. If I didn't have cancer, I would have been complaining about school lunches too. It was just hard for me to make small talk and relate to those who weren't going through what I was in the moment. In the previous chapter, I mentioned that I found myself isolating at times, and this was part of the reason; it was just too emotionally exhausting to be around people who didn't understand.

Blocking out Negativity

Even worse than being around people who don't understand are the negative Nancies; you know who I am talking about. These are the people who tell you how sorry they are for what you are going through and then follow it up with how many people they know who died from the same disease. This used to make me very angry. I didn't want to hear about people dying; I wanted to hear about the woman who survived and lived a long, cancer-free life.

After it happened time after time, I realized I had to change my perspective on this if I was going to maintain my sanity. I recognized that when people tell me about their loved one who died, it's not about the loved one;

it's about them. They are trying to connect on a deeper level, and this is the way they know how. These people are looking for commonality and using the passing of their loved one to cultivate empathy. I try to make sure I show empathy back and tell them I am sorry for their loss, which usually ends the conversation.

If the conversation doesn't end, and the negativity continues, I politely explain that I am currently healthy and cancer-free, and I don't want to talk or think about anything negative about it at the time. It's good to have a line or two to deliver with love when you feel overcome by someone's negative stories or life experiences. This helps set the boundaries around what you will let in and what you won't. Immersing yourself back into your community after cancer isn't easy. This is the time when boundaries are incredibly important and also a time in which you may choose to confide in some people close to you about your struggles. Do it at your own pace, don't be afraid to ask for help, and remember that perspective is everything.

Finding Like-Minded People

About seven months before I was diagnosed, I got a call from a fellow photographer named Liz. Liz was just about thirty years old, was diagnosed with breast cancer, and was about to undergo a bilateral mastectomy. She asked me if I could fit her in for a pre-surgical photo shoot so she could remember what her body and her breasts looked like before her surgery. I told her that I would, of course, make room for her in my schedule. She asked what I charge, and I explained that I didn't want money to be a factor in deciding if she wanted this shoot or not, so I would do it no charge, under one condition. The one condition was that she pay it forward to someone else one day when they needed it most. She agreed.

Liz's photo shoot was a beautiful experience. We laughed; we cried. She had her hair and makeup done and dressed in a beautiful wardrobe. The experience gifted her moments of beauty, normalcy, and fun – moments in which she could forget about doctor's appointments and insurance issues. I worked with cancer patients before, but something about Liz hit a chord in me. As an empath, I felt her struggle deeply. I was trying to put myself in her shoes. For days, I remember thinking, *what would I do if I was told I had to remove my breasts? How would that feel emotionally and physically?* I work with a lot of women going through all sorts of struggles, but for some reason, Liz lived in my heart and on my mind for some time.

Fast forward seven months, and my diagnosis came, and who do you think I called? My parents, of course – but my second call was to Liz. I said, "Liz, I am sorry to bother you, but I was diagnosed with breast cancer, and I don't know what to do."

Without hesitation, Liz sprang into action. She told me who to call and how to organize my papers and doctor's appointments. She assured me that I was going to be okay and that I had a friend in her whenever I needed it. Liz might not know this, but she talked me off many ledges during my treatment.

About a week before my surgery, I got a text from Liz asking if she could come over to drop off some things for me. When she arrived, she had a huge bag of items to help me with my post-surgery life. Then, she asked me if I wanted to see her breasts – and yes, I did! Up until that point, all I had seen online were before/ after photos that scared the hell out of me. Allowing me to see her chest, providing me with comfort items for my surgery, and knowing that I had Liz's support was incredibly comforting during an uncomfortable time. Comforting me and providing me with the items I needed was her way of paying it forward to me. To this day, the irony of that experience still gives me the chills.

These stories remind me how important it is to be surrounded by like-minded people during your treatment, but especially as you put your life back together. Let's face it, no matter the quality or quantity of the support around you, no one quite understands you like another survivor.

Choosing Your Community

There are a plethora of options for community post-breast cancer. My recommendation is to choose wisely. When I looked for support, I first turned to Facebook groups. There were so many groups geared towards breast cancer, and I feverishly joined as many as I could – big mistake. Most of the groups were filled with women who were truly suffering. There were lots of photos of botched surgeries, burnt skin from radiation, and story after story of tragedy. It terrified me. I started to wonder if that was the only option for life after breast cancer – a life of pain and tragedy.

I decided to stop checking the groups because I wanted to make sure I maintained positivity. I realized that the women who struggled were home and connected through social media, but the women who were doing well and feeling positive were too busy for Facebook. They were out living life!

Everyone has a different way of connecting with community after going through this experience. Some women run races, some help with fundraising, and others start businesses to serve the community – there are a million ways to connect! Personally, I connected by making my videos and adding to my YouTube channel when I could. This allowed me to start networking and meeting women who lived beautiful lives and showed cancer who was boss. As a photographer and storyteller, I always look for the story behind the person. The more survivors I met, the more I photographed and talked to them, and the more I realized that the women who were living their lives still suffered from many of the things I suffered with at one point or another. That was when I decided to write this book and create a space on Facebook for positivity. The community I was looking for was one that I needed to create.

It's okay to need support after you are done with treatment and even for years to come. In fact, cancer has brought some of the most incredible women into my life who I wouldn't have met otherwise. You can find support based on need or common interests. Just remember, if you are struggling with something, chances are someone else is too. We don't have to be alone in this fight.

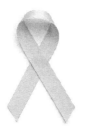

Chapter 14:
Obstacles to Normalcy

"Obstacles do not block the path; they are the path."
— Anonymous

14

Throughout the book so far, I have taken you on a journey to help identify and change the areas in your life that will lead to reconstructing your new normal post-cancer. It's a process that is filled with excitement, joy, and an abundance of self-discovery. You want change. You need change. You have committed to digging your heels into the process. I applaud you! As usual, I am also going to be honest with you. You are human. To be human means there is going to be struggle. Obstacles will appear and try to veer you off course. This chapter is about supporting you through those obstacles and reminding you, this is not a sprint. It's a marathon.

In Chapter 12, I introduced you to the Abraham-Hicks Emotional scale. Here is it again for reference:

1. JOY/APPRECIATION/EMPOWERED/FREEDOM/LOVE
2. PASSION
3. ENTHUSIASM/EAGERNESS/HAPPINESS

4. POSITIVE EXPECTATION/BELIEF

5. OPTIMISM

6. HOPEFULNESS

7. CONTENTMENT

8. BOREDOM

9. PESSIMISM

10. FRUSTRATION/IRRITATION/IMPATIENCE

11. OVERWHELM

12. DISAPPOINTMENT

13. DOUBT

14. WORRY

15. BLAME

16. DISCOURAGEMENT

17. ANGER

18. REVENGE

19. HATRED/RAGE

20. JEALOUSY

21. INSECURITY/GUILT/UNWORTHINESS

22. FEAR/GRIEF/DEPRESSION/DESPAIR/POWERLESSNESS

I mentioned how we could run the range of emotions daily (sometimes even hourly), but there is something I noticed about this scale that was interesting to me. It seems to me that the scale also represents the emotions we experience from the minute we are diagnosed until the present. No matter where you are on your journey, I think it's safe to say that on day one, we were all at fear, grief, and despair. (twenty-two) The question is, how far have you moved up the scale since then?

Personally, I moved up the scale quite a bit, only to be knocked down again when treatment was over. There's no shame in that. This is a fluid process, but I had a decision to make, and now you do too. Where on the scale do you want to live? Do you want to survive cancer only to find that you are now living in anger, worry, frustration, and pessimism, or do you want to live a life filled with optimism, happiness, passion, and joy? Since you are reading this book, I know you are choosing the latter. I did too, but it isn't always easy. Let's talk about some obstacles that can get in your way.

Obstacles and How to Combat Them

To be alive is to face adversity; this process is no exception. As much as we crave change, change can also be scary. No doubt, putting your life back together after cancer means you will experience so many beautiful things. It also means you will face some difficult things. For example, you might want to leave a job or a relationship that never fulfilled you. Maybe you want to do something big, like move across the country, or something smaller, like cutting red meat out of your diet. Big or small, change can be uncomfortable and challenging.

Often, people around you won't understand you and your new perspective on life. You are a different person than you were before in a lot of ways, and that makes others uncomfortable. That might put some strain on your relationships, which is difficult and might lead you to question yourself and fall back into old habits.

Falling back into old habits and thoughts is to be expected and is normal. That is what we call the "comfort zone." Our bodies and minds tend to want to live in the comfort zone, not always because it's what makes us happy, but because it doesn't cause pain and discomfort. That's why they call it the *comfort zone*.

This is the time to get real with yourself. The truth is, there is discomfort in both staying in your comfort zone and stepping outside of it. So, the real question is, which is more uncomfortable for you right now – staying in your comfort zone and living a life that feels foreign, being numb from your feelings, and lacking happiness and joy, or stepping outside your comfort zone and embracing the pain of pushing through your boundaries, which will lead to finding happiness and joy on the other side? If you aren't sure, I will leave this quote right here to help you out:

> *"Life begins at the end of your comfort zone."*
> *– Neale Donald Walsch*

I love to challenge myself to step outside my comfort zone. I try to identify the things in life that I convinced myself are too hard for me, and then I tackle them. Sometimes I take on a big challenge, like running a half marathon (at the time, I couldn't even run down the street without losing my breath!). Sometimes stepping out of my comfort zone is posting topless, post-surgical photos of myself (every time I do, I hold my breath). 30-day challenges are one of my favorite quick and easy ways to push myself. In the past, I have given up chocolate for a month, gone vegan, walked 15,000 steps a day, whatever it is that I don't necessarily think I can do, or even want to do, I do it!

Although these examples are all fun, not all of my stepping out of my comfort zone was rainbows and unicorns. After cancer, I realized that my marriage had taken a big hit. Maybe it was because I had changed or because it was just a lot for a couple to deal with, I don't really know the answer. What I did know was that my relationship wasn't bringing me joy, and I had to be honest about it. It was an incredibly difficult challenge to face. There was a lot of self-doubt and confusion. My mind was telling me that I was going crazy, and I should shut my mouth and not rock the boat. But my heart and my gut nagged me. They told me that if I was to live a healthy, joyful life, I needed to be honest with my partner and myself. Being honest with him was the hardest thing I have ever done. It was also the best. It has opened up our lines of communication. It has allowed me to set boundaries. It has helped us work through a plentitude of issues that most couples have but never tackle. Once I did that, I knew I could do anything.

Stepping out of your comfort zone changes your brain. It proves to it that you can do hard things. When you have moments that you feel like giving up, your brain reminds you that you have done hard things before, and you can do it again. When tackling challenging things head-on, you are creating opportunities for growth. Opportunities for growth bring you closer to every positive emotion you want to experience on a daily basis. This is one of the areas you don't have to surrender to. Don't wait for opportunity to come knocking, be a badass, and create your own path to growth.

Creating the Life You Crave

In Chapter 6, you learned about surrendering the things you don't have control over in your life to a higher power. As I mentioned before, it is the exact opposite. Now is the time to take the bull by the horns and take control of what you can! Cancer has made us feel powerless. There is no arguing that, but here's a news-flash for you, it's a trap! It's a story you are telling yourself. You, my dear, are NOT powerless. In fact, now that you have gone through something incredibly challenging, you are more powerful than ever. It's time to tap into that resource of bountiful energy. This is your life and your creation; it's a blank canvas, and you are the artist. As an artist myself, I adore that analogy. I think it applies in so many ways. When I used to draw and paint, there were times I looked at a blank canvas, and I would immediately get to work, knowing what I wanted it to look like. Those times were rare. Most times, I stared at the canvas for hours without any direction. It felt overwhelming just to take the first step. Sometimes, I would experience both simultaneously! I knew what I wanted the painting to look like, but I didn't know how to create it, so I was frozen.

Sometimes, I could create on my own, and sometimes I needed help. Those were the times I looked outside myself for inspiration and direction, searching on Pinterest or Instagram. I signed up for a class or connected with other artists.

Reconstructing your life after cancer works the same way. You have three options:

- Do it on your own
- Do it with outside support
- Any combination of the two

For me, there are very few challenges in life that I have tackled without someone by my side. I love the companionship and the accountability. I often attempt my 30-day challenges with a friend. When I trained for my half marathon, I hired a coach to make sure I was doing it correctly. When I sat for chemotherapy, having a loved one by my side always made the time go by more quickly.

There is no one roadmap to a joyful life. Just like all women and their breast cancer journeys are unique, so are the ways we reconstruct our lives. One of the hurdles that we all face as humans is that we can't always see our given potential. There's an expression that says, "You can't read the label from the inside of the bottle," and this explains why it is so difficult for us to see our situations and ourselves objectively and why it's great to have help along the way.

In addition to not being able to see ourselves objectively, we are on a constant path of growth and change. Life moves quickly, which forces us to constantly reassess where we currently are and what will move us up on the scale to our desired emotion and life. This is going to be an ongoing process filled with obstacles. The more you do it, the better you will get at it. Just like when I create art, there are times when I can tackle it on my own with minor resistance. The majority of the time, I recognized that having outside help and support has given me a greater understanding of myself and created a solid foundation for change. It has made the process of stepping outside my comfort zone less painful and allows me to move up the scale with greater ease.

There is no right or wrong way to reconstruct your life. You have a blank canvas in front of you. The most important take away I hope you get from this chapter is that you know there will be obstacles you have to overcome, but they don't stop you from taking action. Keep putting one foot in front of the other, day-by-day. I am a true believer in presence over perfection. Stop aiming for perfection and just be present in your life and in this process. Remember obstacles don't block the path, they are the path.

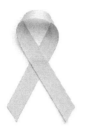

Chapter 15:
Life Begins Today

"My life didn't please me, so I created my life."
— Coco Chanel

15

When I was diagnosed with cancer, I immediately knew that there had to be a bigger purpose in this for me. Right before my diagnosis, I remember praying to the universe, asking how I could reach more women. I kept saying, "Universe, help me reach and help more women. Show me the way." Well, I learned that the way I think it should go and the way it often goes can be two different things.

When I was diagnosed, I often wondered if I actually manifested my cancer; if I did, why did the universe choose to deliver this way as the way to reach more women? I am not sure I will ever have an answer to that. Regardless, I felt it in every bone in my body that I had to make my experience available to as many people as I could.

Going public with my experience with cancer gave my disease purpose. Without purpose, it's just sickness.

Who on earth wants sickness? No one – but we *all* want purpose!

I took to Facebook and made my first video. I spoke about how I found my cancer and how I was going to have a double mastectomy. The video got more views than any video I ever made. It was a little tap on my shoulder from the universe, confirming I was doing the right thing.

After I had my mastectomy, I made at least one video a week. I talked about the healing process, my feelings, expanders, and the struggles. My audience came along and supported me every step of the way.

Then I went through reconstruction, and I spoke about that. I shared photos of my breasts; I talked about the things no one else talked about. I built a community around me that helped me stay positive and heal. It was an outlet for me too. When I couldn't tell my loved ones what was going on in my mind and heart, I was still able to express it in a video.

Then, one day I turned the camera on myself and started healing through self-portraits. I showed the world what a woman without breasts looked like. I tried to show the beautiful side of being a survivor – the strong side. I tried to make the side that is normally terrifying approachable and artistic, and at the same time, somewhat disarming and shocking.

What I didn't realize was that I was also looking for ways to heal. I didn't know that when you are diagnosed with cancer, you can't process it. You can't mourn. You don't worry about missing your breasts.

You are told you will die if you don't remove the cancer, so you strap on that hospital gown, lay yourself on the gurney, and ask them to remove your breasts. Personally, it wasn't until treatment was over that I could even process what happened. I mean, I was in survival mode – hardcore! When your life is threatened, you don't think; you just react. When the war is over, that is when you ask yourself – *what the hell just happened? What did I do?*

This experience is a little shocking, actually, and even more shocking is that everyone around us has had time to process it. They have accepted it and worked through it. In that way, we are so far behind. We are just first getting a chance to look in the mirror and be with ourselves, dealing with the loss, the scare, the physical changes, the mental impact, the PTSD, the confusion, the why me questions, the horror, the fear, the scars, etc.

It's so ironic, isn't it? At the exact moment you think you are going to get your life back, it first hits you that you are falling apart and that you don't recognize your life as it is. You are changed; I was changed – massively. When I thought I was going to get my life back together, it became apparent that I was a giant mess. I wrote this book two years after my treatment ended, and as I wrote it, I was still in the process of figuring it all out. I thought I was going to be one of those patients who just bounced back from chemo and surgery, ran a marathon, lost twenty pounds, and was positive thinking all the time.

I was shocked and disappointed (and sometimes still am) that it wasn't as easy as I thought it was going to be. I felt all sorts of shame. I felt horrible that I wasn't happy about being alive. There were people out there in way worse shape than I was. Why couldn't I find my gratitude? Where was my positive thinking? What was wrong with me?

I searched for other women who struggled with life after cancer. I went to support groups on Facebook, but as I mentioned, those were filled with misery and fear. I tried to talk to friends and family, but they just didn't get it. They tried, but the truth is, unless you have been through it, it's impossible to understand truly.

That was when I knew I had to write this book, just like I knew I had to make the videos in the beginning. Once again, I knew that if I needed this, so many women out there needed it too. I know women need support after their journey to help them reconstruct their lives and find a new normal, and in that, I built a community of like-minded women who don't just want to be alive but want to *feel* alive.

You are one of those women; I wrote this book for you. I wrote this book to heal and document my journey, and I wrote this book to leave a legacy and turn my damn disease into a purpose way bigger than myself. I wrote this book because it is needed. I wrote this book because breast cancer is becoming more and more widespread. I also wrote this book to help support women of the sandwich generation. The sandwich generation refers to people in their thirties and forties who are responsible for both the caretaking of their children and their aging parents. We are incredibly busy taking care of everyone else, but let's be honest, someone needs to take care of us, too. I wrote this book because I thought I couldn't, and now knowing I can means that I can tackle a lot of other things in life that I think I can't do. I know you; I see you. I know you can do hard things too.

Everything you have been through in life and cancer has brought you to this moment. Now I turn the process over to you. You are the artist of your life. You are equipped with the tools you need to reconstruct and live your greatest life. It's time to pick up the toolbox and get to work. Every day that you are given the gift of opening your eyes is an opportunity to start, to make a change, to be different.

My wish for you, dear reader and fellow warrior, is that this book helps you identify the emotional, physical, and spiritual gaps in your life and create a road map on how to realign them so you can redefine and reconstruct your new post-cancer normal, allowing you to take care of yourself fully, increase your self-worth, and live a joyful life, in which you are truly alive.

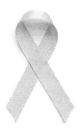

Photo Gallery

Although this book isn't about the details of my medical journey, I wanted to take an opportunity to share some images that I took over the last three years that show a bit of what I went through. It was virtually impossible to pick 20(ish) images that could sum up the magnitude of my experience.

If you want to see more images, please follow me at www.instagram.com/JenRozenbaum

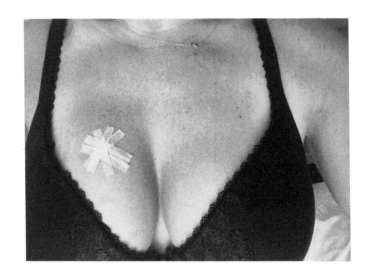

July 10, 2017.

The day I got my sonogram and biopsy.
I had no idea what was in store for me.

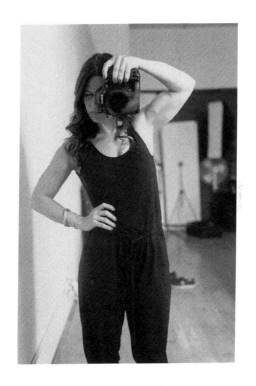

July 11, 2017.

Selfie in my photography studio.
Taking a photo, wondering when my doctor
would call and what I would hear.

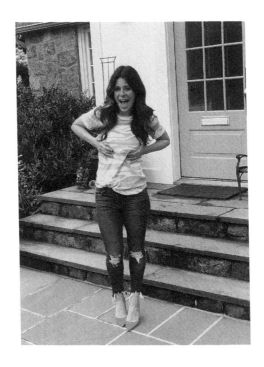

August 2, 2017.

The morning of my mastectomy.
I chose my outfit carefully.
Camo shirt (ready for war) and
pink suede Manolo Blahnik heels.

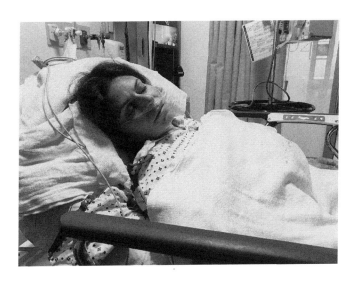

August 2, 2017.

After nine hours the surgery is done.

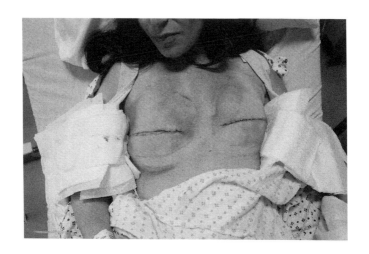

August 3, 2017.

This is the first photo of my new chest.
My Doctor took this photo at my request.
I immediately felt pride in my scars.

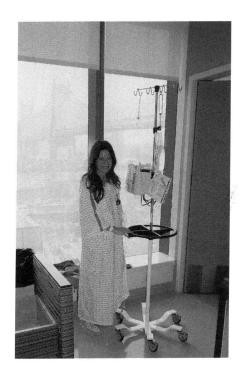

August 3, 2017.

Finally able to stand and move
around it was time to go home.

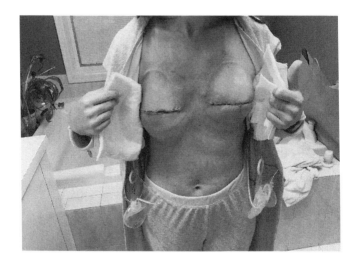

Finally home. I took a photo almost
every day to track my healing.

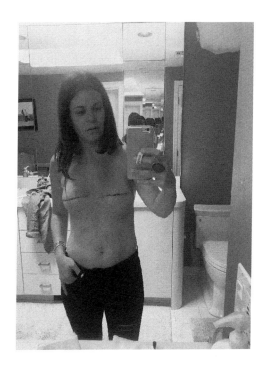

A few weeks after surgery I finally have
my drain removed and I start getting my
tissue expanders filled little by little.

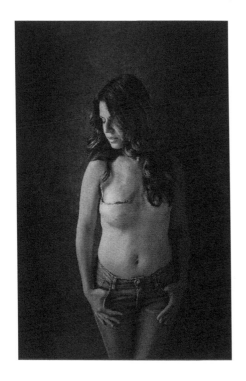

Done with my tissue expander fills.
I look deformed but it doesn't matter.
It's part of my journey and I wanted to
remember it. *(Photo credit to my girl Seely.)*

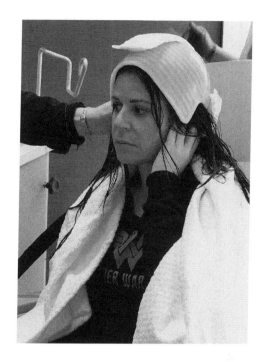

September 18, 2017.

I start 8 rounds of CMF Chemotherapy.
I used a cold cap to save my hair.

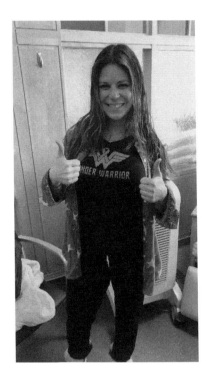

December 27, 2017.

Done with Chemotherapy and
ready for a new year to roll in.

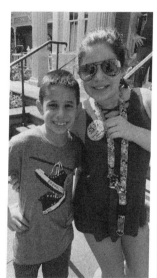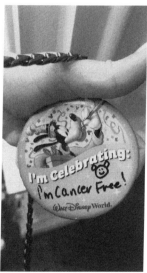

February 2018.

Off to Disney with the family to
celebrate life and being cancer free!

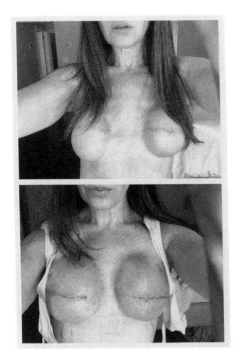

March 15, 2018.

Before/After – Tissue Expanders to Implants.
How ridiculous do my tissue expanders look?
I was relieved to get rid of them.

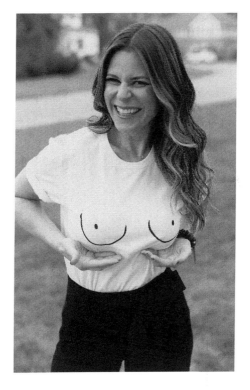

Sometimes I keep my shirt on ;)

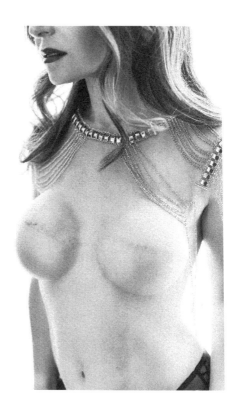

October 17, 2018.

In an effort to embrace my new body,
I have boudoir photos taken by Kara Marie.

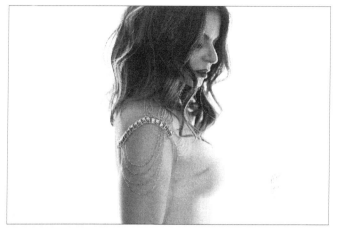

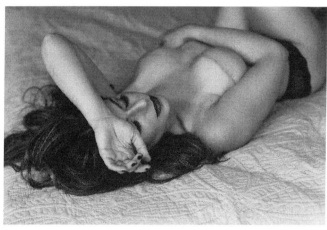

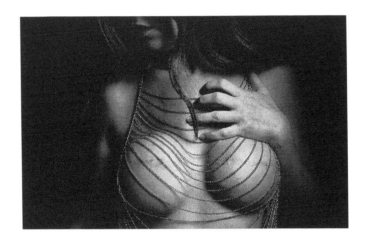

During my journey I have turned the
camera on myself many times. Photography
is part of my healing and acceptance.

JEN ROZENBAUM

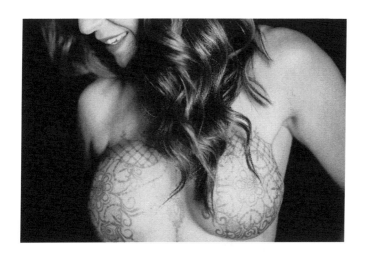

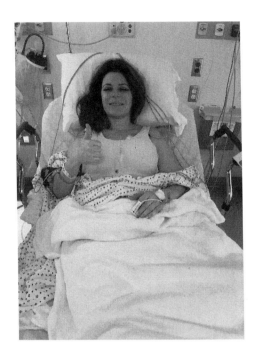

November 7, 2019.

My second attempt at reconstruction
surgery after my first one looked horrible.
Unfortunately this surgery didn't look good
either and I needed another reconstruction.

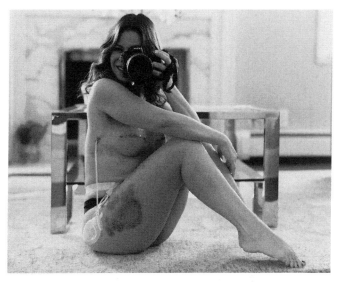

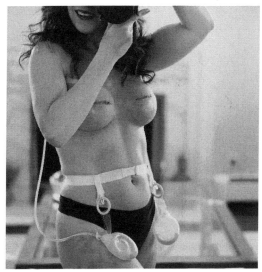

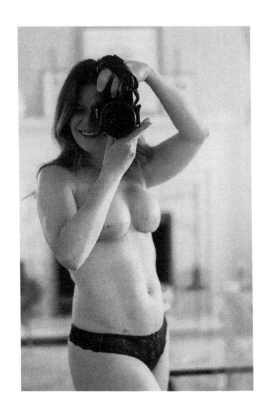

July 15, 2020.

One week after my third
reconstruction surgery.

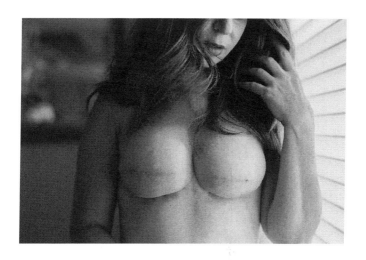

Acknowledgements

When I was eighteen years old, I was out with some friends for dinner. There was a psychic at the restaurant that night, and just for kicks, we all signed up to get a reading from her. To this day, I couldn't tell you anything she said, except for this one piece of information that always stuck with me.

She told me I was going to write a book one day. I am not sure why I remember that. I never considered myself a writer, and I had no idea what I would write about, but the idea of doing something so tremendous and out of my comfort zone always appealed to me.

I have my parents to thank for that. They always taught me, "If it was easy, anyone could do it!" Little did I know, those words would sculpt me into the person I am and got me through the hardest times in my life. I always said that the only thing worse than getting cancer is having a child with cancer. Even though I was forty-one at the time of diagnosis, I know that I am still my parents' baby, at any age. Mom *and* Dad, I want to thank you for your love, support, babysitting, phone calls, meals, and unconditional love always, but especially for your support through my cancer journey. I know I wasn't the only one suffering, and it was incredibly hard on you too, yet you stood by my side every single moment.

To my dear children Talia and Sam, the last thing I ever wanted in life was for you to experience a sick mother. It broke my heart every day. The fact that I didn't have the energy to make you dinner or that I had to rush bedtime so I could go to sleep just scratches the surface of what cancer has robbed from me, and from you. My hope for you, my loves, is that this experience contributes to you being the most empathetic people. I hope I modeled for you how to handle struggle with a sense of hope and that one day when you struggle in your life, you too will know that you are strong enough to get through it. I hope one day you will look back and know that your love carried me through every minute of every day. Most of all, I want you to know that I am proud of you and I love you more than words can ever express. You are my world.

To Micha, from day one, you swooped in and took on so much. You were often the roles of Mom and Dad. You packed lunches, picked up from school, and made sure I was comfortable and taken care of through treatment and surgery. You occupied the kids, helped me with my physical therapy, and hugged me when I cried. I am grateful to you for that.

To Jason, Kristin, Axel, Chanan, Mim, Jonah, and Lyla, you are the best brothers, sisters, nieces, and nephews I could ask for, and I love you all. Thank you for helping my family and me get through this time. Your calls, visits, meals, gifts, thoughts, and prayers will never be forgotten. I hope you know that no matter what happens, I've got your back just as you had mine. M – special shout out to all the tears we have shed together. I keep those conversations close to my heart.

To Susan and Serge, thank you for treating me as one of your own. Your concern, help with the kids, gifts, and love got me through many difficult days. Thank you also for supporting Micha so he could support me. It takes a village to get through times like this.

To Willie and Tex, the two pups that curled up to me and cuddled with me and watched over me as I was healing, thank you. You have proven to me that puppy love is medicine.

To my friends, extended family and my community, both in-person and on social media. Wow. The way you all showed up to support me was beyond my wildest imagination. I was overwhelmed with emails, messages, gifts, prayers, meals, offers of help, and more. I shed happy tears daily. As I was going through the hardest time in my life, it was also the time I felt the most gratitude and connection. I felt every hug, prayer, and good thought run through my body every day.

A few special mentions:

MB and SP, cancer is the 238147387584th hard thing we have all been through together. You are not just friends, you are my family. I am blessed to have you by side and honored to always be by yours.

RO, From the minute I was diagnosed, you put on a cape and became my superhero. You always knew what I needed, even before I did. You made me feel loved like a sister. I will never know how to repay you for what you did for me. Well, maybe I'll start with some snacks.

To AD and LT – We couldn't be more different but

we are connected in every way. That is what I love about us. I felt you hold my hand from afar every moment.

SP – Thank you for being a shining example of what a warrior is. I am lucky to have you in my life and by my side.

To my Israeli Family in Roslyn who cooked, called and cooked some more, I appreciate you taking care of my family, filling their bellies and filling my heart.

Carmit R., Seely, Kara Marie, and Dixie, thank you for helping me heal and capturing my journey through your lenses. It was an experience I will forever remember.

To the unicorns, those once in a lifetime people I have met that believe in me, see me and support me; I am forever indebted to you.

Thank you to Professor Alex and my Muay Thai wifey, Alyssa. You both push me to work hard, teach me discipline and even let me punch and kick you now and again. Muay Thai is fun, but you make it amazing!

To my work family, your support through this meant the world to me. I know you could have easily replaced me with someone who was able to do the job way better than I could, but you never turned your backs on me. In fact, you believed in me and gave me the push I needed to keep at it even in my darkest time. A special thank you to Nikon, Westcott, Fundy, WHCC, and Rangefinder/ WPPI who have not only supported me but given me an outlet to help share my work and raise breast cancer awareness. You truly are all family.

Thank you to Alexa Bigwarfe from "Write Publish Sell" and Liz Thompson from 'House Style Editing'. Your guidance, accountability, brains and love helped me and is going to help so many women. Thank you for helping me get this book out into the world.

Thank you to my team of Doctor's at Memorial Sloan Kettering and NYBRA, who have taken me apart and put me back together. You saved my life, and I will be eternally grateful for that.

Thank you to the breast cancer community. Each and every woman I have met in this journey has touched my heart and soul. I hate cancer, but I am so grateful that it has brought all of you into my life. My life is richer and fuller because of it.

I know cancer stories don't always have happy endings. I am so grateful mine did. Thank you to the universe and the powers that be that allowed me a second chance at life and inspired me to write this book. I am forever grateful to be guided and protected by you.

About the Author

Jen Rozenbaum is a born and bred New Yorker, portrait photographer, and breast cancer survivor. Through her work, both with her camera and without, she is helping women celebrate their unique femininity and helping breast cancer patients and survivors put their lives back together after cancer.

Jen picked up a camera for the first time in 2008 as a tool of healing. She was suffering from fertility issues and turned to photography as a distraction. She spent countless hours teaching herself photography, and in 2009 started a boudoir photography business in her home.

Through her years of photographing women, she learned so much about them and the struggles they go through, whether it be fertility, aging, divorce, motherhood or health issues, Jen helped heal her clients one-by-one by giving them a safe space to express and celebrate their unique femininity. In turn, her clients also healed her by showing her real-life examples of triumph and strength.

Out of her photography work, the Shamelessly Feminine® movement was born, and her work became a mission to empower and heal women across the globe. Jen knew that the more women she could reach, the more the world would change for the better.

Jen was recognized in the photography industry as a leader in the boudoir genre and traveled the globe to share her wealth of knowledge and love for empowering and transforming women. The more she could teach other photographers, the more women could be reached collectively. This is the first time she learned that out of tragedy, something beautiful could be born.

In 2017, when Jen was diagnosed with breast cancer, she instantly knew this was once again an opportunity to turn tragedy into triumph. She made a video announcing her breast cancer that received a lot of attention because it was real, raw, and honest. Since then, Jen has been making videos for her YouTube channel, offering her honest thoughts about topics rarely spoken about around breast cancer.

Her willingness to share her triumphs, struggles, and honest feelings help educate and inspire breast cancer patients and survivors every day. After getting many messages from women after they watched her videos, Jen once again knew that she could serve her community by writing this book and addressing the realities of life after cancer.

Jen lives on Long Island with her two kids, and the cutest rescue pup around. She lives with gratitude every day that she survived cancer and was given a second chance at life. She believes that when playing truth or dare, you should always choose dare, in buying good shoes if you plan to land on your feet, and in trusting your gut – it's always right.

Website:
www.jenrozenbaum.com

Email:
jenrozenbaum@gmail.com

YouTube:
www.youtube.com/jenrozenbaum

Thank You

Thank you so much for reading, *What the F*ck Just Happened?: A Survivors Guide to Life After Breast Cancer.* If you've made it this far, I know one of two things about you. First, you're more ready than ever to create a beautiful life post-breast cancer, and second, maybe you also read the last page the book before diving in – no judgments here!

Connection is so important on this journey. I would love to get to know you better and learn more about your breast cancer journey, so please keep in touch!

You can find me at:

Instagram:
www.instagram.com/jenrozenbaum

Private Facebook group:
(where there is more info about my group mentoring sessions):
https://www.facebook.com/groups/LifeAfterBreast-
CancerwithJenRozenbaum/

YouTube:
https://www.youtube.com/c/jenrozenbaum

and of course at
www.jenrozenbaum.com